Healing

What God Has Provided for His Children

Alta Ada Williams

with

Bruce Williams

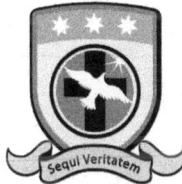

Sequi Veritatem

Lititz Institute
Publishing Division

Published by Lititz Institute Publishing Division
P.O. Box 7808, Lancaster, PA 17604-7808
www.lititzinstitute.org

Printed in the United States of America

Library of Congress Cataloging-in-Publication Data

Williams, Alta Ada.
    Healing: What God Has Provided for His Children /
    Alta Ada Williams.

            p.   cm.

    ISBN 978-0-9820014-1-7   (paperback)

    1. Doctrine of Healing. 2. Methods that God uses for
        healing. 3. Problems and questions about healing.
        I. Title.

All Scripture quotations are taken from The Authorized King James Version of the Holy Bible.

To Bruce, my husband—who has helped me tremendously in my walk with the Lord, who has helped in the writing of this book, and who has shared the life we have in the Lord

Table of Contents

Section III

Section IV

Note:

This book is not intended to take the place of treatment or advice from your physicians. The author does not take any responsibility for any possible consequences from action taken as a result of your reading this book. If you are taking prescription medications, you should consult with your doctor and go off the medications only with the supervision of your doctor. In the book we relate the story of individuals who turned down medical treatment when they thought they were healed, with disastrous results.

Introduction

In 1995 both Bruce and I received healing for physical problems that were supposedly "incurable." We were very thankful to the Lord. We can still remember the excitement at being relatively pain free for the first time in years. (We relate parts of my story throughout the book, and Bruce tells his story in Chapter 7.)

This healing was consistent with our faith. We had always believed that God *could* heal "when it was His will," and we were so very grateful that He had chosen to heal us. We did not understand that God *always* wants to heal and that part of His character is being the Healer.

Our interplay with God's healing had begun years before. When I was a child, my mother came very close to death; and my father and mother always attributed her healing to God's intervention. A very close prayer partner and friend of mine had been miraculously healed more than forty years ago from terminal illness (we tell Susan's story in Chapter 6). I had read and reread her testimony and always was thrilled to know how gracious God was to her in healing her. These examples reinforced to me that God *could* heal "if it was His will."

When Bruce was in his final year of medical school, he became a believer. Shortly thereafter, he read a book by a Scottish physician who had the gift of healing. Bruce thought that was a wonderful combination—to be trained in medicine and also to have the gift of healing. He asked God at that time to give him the gift of healing. Soon afterward, Bruce was involved in churches that downplayed healing at the very least; and this prayer lay dormant for more than 20 years.

In 1993 he prayed for healing for me on one occasion with success, but we thought it was "just" the answer to that particular prayer. Not until 1995 did Bruce learn that he did indeed have the gift of healing. And not until the late 1990's did we understand that any believer can pray for healing for another believer and that God will answer that prayer (see discussion in Chapter 6).

In 1995, as a result of our healing, we began to look at some of the Scriptures dealing with healing again. At one point we were each looking at Isaiah 53 independently of each other. We knew that the "charismatics" taught that the passage "with his stripes we are healed" meant physical healing, while the more fundamentalist groups taught that this healing was partial at best in this life and would be complete when we get our resurrection bodies.

During this time Bruce began to sense that healing was probably available in the atonement, but I told Bruce one day, "Nothing can ever make me believe that healing is in the atonement and available for all believers." I believed that the teaching that all believers could be healed—or that healing is in the atonement—was heresy. I felt that it had falsely raised the hopes of many people. In fact, I had had a friend who died, saying, "If I could only have had more faith, I could have been healed." It seemed to me that this idea made healing man's work, and this further prejudiced me against believing in healing for all believers.

Bruce had been prejudiced by some experiences. On one occasion he had a diabetic patient tell him that she had been healed in a "healing service" and that she would no longer take her insulin. Sadly, a few years later she returned to his office with a gangrenous leg. The gangrene developed because she had not been healed, and diabetes out of control can cause gangrene. The leg had to be amputated. Thus, he was skeptical at the very least of "faith healings."

Nevertheless, we continued to study God's Word. We strongly felt (and still do) that we should base every doctrine on the Word of God, and we had always been willing to be shown some new truth from the Word. We wanted to know what God's Word teaches on healing. With this background we tackled this doctrine head-on. I asked God Himself to show me what He means in the Isaiah 53 passage. Chapter 2 deals with this passage in detail, but here I will simply describe my breakthrough in understanding.

I got a hint of the meaning of this passage from a couple of authors I was reading, but the breakthrough came as I looked at some of the words in the original Hebrew language. The KJV reads in verses 4 and 12: "Surely he hath borne our griefs, and carried our sorrows. ... he bare the sin of many."

The word translated "grief" in vs. 3, 4, and 10 is really a word that is usually translated "sickness" (see discussion in Chapter 2). But the real "clincher" is the word translated "borne" and "bare" in vs. 4 and 12. It is the same word in the two verses and is the same word as the one used in Leviticus 16:22 to describe the scapegoat, who bore and carried away the sin of the people. *It is used for atonement.* This passage in Isaiah uses the same word for Christ's bearing our sicknesses and bearing our sin. It goes against all rules of grammar and linguistic interpretation to have the word figurative in one sentence and literal in another unless the passage clearly indicates that fact.

Something "clicked" in my spirit in faith when I realized that the same word is used for the sacrificial scapegoat and for Jesus' bearing our sins and for bearing our illnesses. *There seemed no other way around the truth that He bore our illnesses.*

This study confirmed for Bruce what he was sensing. It is amazing to us that, out of all the myriad of sermons we had heard on this passage, we had never heard anyone deal with these words properly. (We now know that some Bible teachers and ministers do teach this doctrine, but we had not heard it at that time.)

Chapter 2 discusses the implications of this discovery. Here I would just comment that it has deepened our love for the Lord to understand that not only did He bear on the cross every sin but all disease. We cannot comprehend such suffering! What Love! With this breakthrough on understanding God's great healing grace, we found that Scriptures began to open themselves to us. We have been amazed to see that the entire Scriptures abound with the message that our God is truly "Yahweh Rapha," or the "God Who is the Great Healer." It is our desire that this book will help the reader to see the many ways that God does heal and to understand that it is truly God's will that all believers be healed.

The first section will be a rather academic examination of the doctrine of healing. After establishing that part of God's very character is being the Great Healer, we will look at the Biblical basis for healing. We will see that the Bible does teach that healing was provided in the atonement.

The second section will examine the doctrine of healing. We will first see what it is. Then we will discuss how an individual can take the doctrine of healing and apply it. We will develop the faith principle. By using that principle, we will see what is necessary for healing to be efficacious for the believer. We will see how to transfer knowledge of healing into actual healing. Finally, we will discuss the counterattacks to healing.

The third section will look at the many different methods God uses to heal today; this will include examining the spiritual gifts of healing. We will also distinguish between the direct miracle and the use of faith and *rhema* in healing. Much of this section will be anecdotal, as we relate how various people have used "their" *rhema* for healing. Since Bruce's healing covers a number of years and includes many different principles developed in this book, he relates his story in a separate chapter.

The fourth section will deal with problems or questions. We will answer some of the objections to belief in God's healing for today's church. We will answer questions about cases in which God does not heal, and we will give suggestions for personal healing.

Some of the chapters will be fairly academic in order to establish clearly doctrine related to healing. Some of the material is more anecdotal in order to show our journey into understanding of this doctrine and to show how it works in today's world. It is our hope that, by showing part of this as a journey, we will be able to encourage you to make this same journey. When helpful, we have told the story of particular individuals, but we have changed names and certain identifying features of the healings in most cases to protect the privacy of the individuals.

This book assumes that the reader is a believer in the Lord Jesus Christ as Lord and Savior. If you have never encountered the living God and come into a personal relationship with Him, physical illness is not your biggest problem. You need first to meet God in a saving encounter from your sin, and then you can claim his promises for healing. Since it is outside the scope of this book to elaborate on the salvation process, we would just mention a few basic points.

God created the earth and all its inhabitants and pronounced His work "very good" (Genesis 1:31). He gave man free choice, and the first man and woman chose to disobey God's word—thus bringing sin, disease, and death to the entire human race (Genesis 2:16-17; 3:6,14-19; Romans 5:12). Since that time all men have sinned and fall short of God's glory (Romans 3:23). God's great love for us, however, found a way to bridge the chasm that sin had left between Him and us. He provided for God the Son to be born as a man, live a sinless life, and pay the penalty that we ought to pay by His atoning death on the cross. By our acceptance of this sacrifice, we exchange the curse of sin for the blessings obtained for us by His Son Jesus. All of this is succinctly summed up in one verse, Romans 6:23: "For the wages of sin is death, but the gift of God is eternal life through Jesus Christ, our Lord." If you have never prayed, asking God to be your Savior, this is your greatest need. It is our prayer that you will pray this prayer and thus enter the family of God. Then, and then only, will you receive the benefits of sonship, one of which is the right to pray for your healing. Although God can perform a miracle, and sometimes does, by healing an unbeliever, the unbeliever does not have a legal basis on which to seek healing.

For whom, then, have we written this book? We have written primarily for believers, particularly for those believers who are as we were for so many years—that is, believers who believe God *can* heal when He desires but who do not understand that God desires every believer to receive healing. We want you to be released from the confines of having God and His power for you boxed up. We are not writing to convince those who do not believe that we serve a God Who intervenes supernaturally in our lives. Nor are we writing for the theologian. Most theologians who do not believe in God's healing nature know quite well all the arguments from the Bible. They have simply made a choice not to believe. Jesus told us that, after He ascended to His Father and when the Holy Spirit would be poured out on His church, the Holy Spirit would guide the believer into all truth (John 16:13). As a believer, therefore, you should ask the Holy Spirit, Who is resident in you, to enlighten you to the truth as you read the ideas we set forth.

One explanation is necessary concerning a grammatical point. In standard English, pronouns must agree in number and gender with their antecedents. Whenever the gender could be either male or female, standard English uses the male. Thus, the following sentence would be correct: "Each believer must decide for himself what he will do." Since believer is singular and since the gender is not specified, the masculine is used. Modern "politically correct" writers frequently avoid this situation by making the pronoun plural: "Each believer must decide for themselves what they will do." Alternately, some writers use the awkward "Each believer must decide for himself or herself what he or she will do." Neither of these attempts to avoid using the masculine pronoun is acceptable, the former one being incorrect grammar and the latter being very awkward. Thus, in this book we have used the traditional English grammar form, the masculine, when the gender is not specified. Obviously, any statement concerning a believer or an individual should be understood to apply equally to males and females except where context specifically precludes this reading.

All Scriptures are from the Authorized King James Version of The Holy Bible. In the King James Version, when a word is supplied that was not in the original, the translators indicated this fact by putting the word in italics. I have left those in the text; if I add italics, I indicate it.

Section I

1

The Character of God

In order to understand healing, we must first understand something about the character of God. As God began to reveal His character to man historically, He used many ways to do this. All His acts in history from creation to the end of time serve not only to advance His purposes but also to reveal His character. We will look at God's character revealed by His names, God's character revealed in the ministry of Jesus, and God's character revealed in its impartation to believers in the Church Age.

God's Character Revealed by His Names

As God interacted with man and, more particularly, as He interacted with Israel as a nation, He used His names as a revelation of His character. Names in Hebrew were used to indicate character. Thus, God changed Abram's name (meaning "high father") to Abraham (meaning "father of many nations") to indicate the change in the relationship Abraham had with God. Henceforth, he would be a father of many nations; *i.e.*, he would be fulfilling the covenant promise made by God.

God changed Jacob's name (meaning "supplanter") to Israel (meaning "God prevails"). This change indicates the progress made by the man who supplanted his brother Esau by purchasing his birthright and stealing the blessing from his father to the man who fathered the children who would become the heads of the twelve tribes of the nation. In fact, the very nation would take its name, Israel, from this new name. And this nation, Israel, would prevail throughout all history. It would be a sign that God and God's plans do prevail.

One of the most compelling arguments for God as a healer today involves a rather technical study of one of God's names. There are three primary names of God used in the Bible. As these are first revealed in the Old Testament, we will look at them as they are used in the Hebrew. The first name of God used in the Bible is *Elohim*, אֱלֹהִים, (Genesis 1:1). This word comes from a stem meaning "God" but has a plural ending, possibly showing the Trinity in the name. Thus, Genesis 1:26 says: "And God [Elohim] said, Let **us** make man in **our** image, after **our** likeness…" [our emphases].

Another name of God used in the Bible is *Adonai*, אֲדֹנָי, meaning "Lord" or "Master." This word can be used of our Heavenly Lord or an earthly lord—as a king, lord of a manor, master (of a servant), or husband (Sarah called Abraham her lord). The first usage of this word is in Genesis 15:2 as a compound with YHWH. Its first usage by itself is in Genesis 18:3. In that passage Abraham addressed God as though from a servant's position: "…My Lord, if now I have found favor in thy sight, pass not away, I pray thee, from thy servant."

It is the third name of God, YHWH, יְהוָה, (transliterated as Yahweh or Jehovah), however, on which we want to focus our attention. This name was revealed in its fullness to Moses. Although the Bible uses this name before this revelation, God tells Moses that He was not known by this name to Abraham, Isaac, and Jacob (Exodus 6:3). This name was frequently used when God was stressing a covenantal relationahip.

When God appeared to Moses with His commission, Moses asked God, "…when I come unto the children of Israel, and shall say unto them, The God of your fathers hath sent me unto you; and they shall say to me, What is his name? what shall I say unto them?" (Exodus 3:13). God answered him, "I AM THAT

I AM; and he said, Thus shalt thou say unto the children of Israel, I AM hath sent me unto you" (Exodus 3:14).

The word translated "I AM" in the KJV is really untranslatable as a name. The Hebrew language does not have tense in the same way Indo-European languages do. Various stems can be used to show relative time; in actual usage they serve in much the same way tenses do. What God does in the passage above is to use the base word meaning "existence." Since there is not really tense, **God is saying that He is pure existence outside all time constraints**. The word is outside all constraints of time, thus showing the eternality of God. *It is very important for our discussion to understand that this name of God shows eternal existence, outside the boundaries of time, and indicates "to be" or "existence."*

Thus, Jesus' statement, "I am ... the life" takes on much more meaning with this understanding. When Jesus was talking to the Pharisees and mentioned Abraham, He said, "Before Abraham was, I am" (John 8:58). He was assuming the covenant name of God. No wonder the unbelieving leaders wanted to kill Him after that statement. They understood very well that He was claiming to be God.

Similarly, in the garden of Gethsemane, when the soldiers arrived to arrest Jesus, Jesus asked whom they sought. "They answered him, Jesus of Nazareth" (John 17:5) and when Jesus responded, He said, literally, "I am (verse 6—the word *he* is not in the original language)." It was this identification with the name God had revealed to Moses and the power released by the use of this name that caused the soldiers to fall backward to the ground.

In the Old Testament there are many compound names of God (the coupling of two or more of God's names) in addition to the three primary names. These serve to indicate more of God's character. There are at least seven compound names that have as their first name YHWH, the name revealed to Moses and discussed above. (These seven do not count the times YHWH is compounded with one of the other two primary names of God.)

Many of these are well known, and many writings have studied them. "Yahweh tsidkenu" (God is righteousness—Jeremiah 23:6), for example, literally, means "God—personified eternal existence—righteousness." In other words, God, Who personifies eternal existence, eternally exists as righteousness; that is, righteousness is eternally a part of God's character. We do not disregard this revelation of God's character today because it was first revealed in the Old Testament.

Similarly, in Genesis 22:14, the well-known passage recounting when God commanded Abraham to sacrifice Isaac, God reveals Himself as "Yahweh jireh יְהוָה יִרְאֶה" or "God Who sees." There is a word play on the word *see* in the passage. In the chapter, the root word meaning "to see" and, by extension, "to provide" is used in several places. The idea behind the word seems to be that God *sees* something; thus, He *provides* it. This is really talking about looking through the eyes of faith. This word is used several times in Genesis 22. In verse 4b the word is translated *saw*, "…[Abraham] **saw** the place afar off." In verse 8, the same word is translated *provide*: "God will **provide** himself a lamb for a burnt-offering." In verse 13 it is translated *looked,* "Abraham lifted up his eyes, and **looked**…" [emphases ours]. Abraham names the place Jehovahjireh; and Moses, the author of Genesis, remarks that it is known as that to his day and that it means "In the mount of the Lord it shall be seen" (verse 14). The idea is that God "saw to" a sacrifice for Abraham; *i.e.*, he provided it. Abraham had to see it to receive it. The word indicates that it is part of God's eternal character that He provides for His people. New Testament believers have always claimed this provision of God. God never changes; He always provides for His own. David said, "I have been young, and now am old; yet have I not seen the righteous forsaken, nor his seed begging bread" (Psalm 37:25). Paul assures us that "...my God shall supply all your need according to his riches in glory by Christ Jesus" (Philippians 4:19). It is part of God's eternal character that He provides for His children.

In Exodus 15:26 another of these compound names is revealed, "Yahweh rapha רָפָא יְהוָה." These words mean "God Who is the Healer." Once more, the entire construction is such that we are being told that part of God's character is that He is eternally the One Who heals. *Rapha* itself has an active participle construction, indicating that God is always healing. As with the other compound names of God, this name indicates that being the Healer is part of God's unchanging, eternal character.

With the inherent meaning of YHWH one has to break all rules of interpretation to say that God at some point quits healing His people. He is the eternal Healer! If the language alone were not sufficient to show this principle, God reminds us that His character is unchanging. He mentions "Jesus Christ the same yesterday, and to day, and for ever" (Hebrews 13:8). James calls the Lord "the Father of lights, with whom is no variableness, neither shadow of turning" (James 1:17). Malachi quotes God as saying, "For I am the Lord, I change not..." (Malachi 3:6). *Just as "Yahweh tsidkenu" and "Yahweh jireh" still describe God's character today, even so "Yahweh rapha" still describes part of God's character.*

Thus, the first step to understanding God's healing character is to understand that being the Great Healer is part of God's character. This is further borne out in the records of our Lord's ministry.

God's Character Revealed in the Ministry of Jesus

Jesus makes very clear that if one has seen Him, He has seen the Father (John 14:9). The author of Hebrews states that Jesus is "the express image of his [God's] person..." (1:3). Thus, the character of Jesus that we see in the Gospels reveals the character of God. All the Gospels, in their individual ways, show that the healing aspect of the character of God was very active in God, the Son, in His earthly ministry.

There is no recorded instance in which Jesus turned anyone away who asked for healing. In fact, the Synoptic Gospel writers go out of their way to say that Jesus healed *all* who were sick, infirm, or demon possessed. Matthew especially does that. For example, he says, "And Jesus went about *all* the cities and villages, teaching in their synagogues, and preaching the gospel of the kingdom, and healing *every* sickness and *every* disease among the people" (Matthew 9:35—emphases ours). He makes similar statements in several passages: 4:23-24; 8:16-17; 12:15; 14:35-36; and 15:30-31. Other examples in the Synoptic gospels include Mark 1:32-33; Mark 6:55-56; Luke 4:40-41; and Luke 6:19.

John's account is subtler, but just as persuasive when we see the way he organized his gospel. John chooses to recount seven signs, or miracles, that occurred before the resurrection. (He records one that occurred after the resurrection in a chapter that is organized almost as an epilogue to the primary gospel.) These seven signs, around which the gospel is organized, serve to show Jesus as the Son of God. Seven is usually considered the number of completion in Biblical writings; by choosing seven signs, John is showing that this represents a complete picture of Jesus. He chooses three signs to show Jesus' creation powers or powers over the elements of the universe—changing the water into wine; feeding the company of 5000 men, plus women and children; and walking on the water.

The majority (four) of the signs John selects involve healing—healing the nobleman's son, healing the infirm man at the pool of Bethesda, healing the man born blind, and raising Lazarus from the dead. Thus, in a complete picture of Jesus' miracles, more than half are healing miracles. In addition, John, in closing his gospel states, "And many other signs truly did Jesus in the presence of his disciples, which are not written in this book.... And there are also many other things which Jesus did, which, if they should be written every one, I suppose that even the world itself could not contain the books that should be written" (20:30; 21:25). Thus, by implication, the healing ministry of Jesus was extremely big in numbers. It is not surprising that healing plays such an important role in Jesus' ministry, since part of God's character is that He is the Great Healer.

There is another subtle expression of this facet of Jesus' ministry. When a certain leper came to Jesus, we are told that he was "...beseeching him, and kneeling down to him, and saying unto him, If thou wilt, thou canst make me clean. And Jesus, moved with compassion, put forth his hand, and touched him, and saith unto him, I will [lit., am now willing]; be thou clean" (Mark 1:40-41—see also Matthew 8:2-4 and Luke 5:12-14). Jesus tells us that "I came down from heaven, not to do mine own will but the will of him that sent me" (John 6:38). Thus, we know that it was the Father's will to heal the leper. God is willing to heal.

There is one type of exception to the premise that no one in the gospels was ever turned down by Jesus for healing. It is true that the gospels do not record Jesus refusing to heal anyone, but they do record that He was unable to do many miracles, healing included, in certain areas because of unbelief. We deal with unbelief's being an obstacle to healing in more detail in Chapter 6, but we will note two examples here.

Matthew 13:58 and Mark 6:5-6 give us the account of Jesus' last recorded visit to Nazareth, His hometown. There He was rejected; the people did not believe in Him. As a result, He was not able to do many miracles. We are told, "And he did not many mighty works there because of their unbelief" (Matthew 13:58), and "...he could there do no mighty work, save that he laid his hands upon a few sick folks, and healed them" (Mark 6:6).

Even when lack of faith condemned a geographical area, we still see Jesus having compassion and healing individuals. Although Jesus condemned Bethsaida because of its unbelief (Matthew 11:20-24), He still healed the blind man who was brought to Him (Mark 8:22-26). Interestingly, He led the man outside the city (apparently He would not or could not heal in the condemned city); and when He had healed him, He told him neither to go into the town nor to tell it to anyone in the town (verse 26). Thus, even when a geographic area was condemned, Jesus was so much the Great Healer that He healed an individual from that area.

He tested the faith of certain people before He healed, but He did not turn them down. In particular, He did this to Gentiles, as His primary earthly mission before the cross was to offer the kingdom to the Jewish nation. Jesus *appears* to turn down the request of the Syrophenician woman for Jesus to heal her daughter. When Jesus, however, tests her and sees her faith, He tells her that her faith has been responsible for her daughter's healing (Matthew 15:21-28; Mark 7:24-30).

We should never think that Jesus' healing was an automatic action in which He merely applied a formula. The Bible says, for example, that Jesus had to have the power of the Lord in order to heal: "...and the power of the Lord was present for him to heal them" (Luke 5:16). He indicated that sometimes it was not easy at all to heal. When Jesus came down from the Mount of Transfiguration with Peter, James, and John, He discovered that the other disciples had not been able to heal the son of a man in the crowd. After Jesus rebuked the evil spirit and healed the boy, He told His disciples, "This kind can come forth by nothing, but by prayer and fasting" (Mark 9:29). Jesus was referring to prayer and fasting by the one(s) praying for the deliverance.

When Jesus first preached in the synagogue in Nazareth, he quoted from Isaiah 61:1-2 to show that He was the Messiah. He picked a passage that indicates that part of His character is that of the Great Healer, "...he hath anointed me to preach the gospel to the poor; he hath sent me to heal the brokenhearted, to preach deliverance to the captives, and recovering of sight to the blind, to set at liberty them that are bruised" (Luke 4:18).

In addition, when John the Baptist was in prison and sent some of his disciples to ask Jesus if He was, indeed, the Messiah, Jesus told them, "Go your way, and tell John what things ye have seen and heard—how the blind see, the lame walk, the lepers are cleansed, the deaf hear, the dead are raised, to the poor the gospel is preached" (Luke 7:22). Thus He said that He did the works predicted by Isaiah in Chapter 61, which is the passage he had read in the synagogue.

In other words, Jesus' very claim to be One with the Father, the Son of God, was in part predicated on His showing that He, too, is the Great Healer. The gospels, then, are filled with the news that part of Jesus' character, as God Incarnate, is that of the Healer.

There are people who have come to their understanding of the healing nature of God, not by a specific Scripture, but by seeing that this nature is revealed in Jesus as He ministered on earth. Catherine Marshall is one such person.[1]

God's Character Revealed in Its Impartation to Believers in the Church Age

The most amazing aspect of Jesus' healing power is that, as His body, He has given us the same power. *In other words, we share in the very character of God Himself.* That is almost incomprehensible!

First, Jesus empowered the twelve disciples for a specific mission during His earthly ministry: "Then he ... gave them power and authority over all demons, and to cure diseases. And he sent them to preach the kingdom of God, and to heal the sick" (Luke 9:1-2; cp. Matthew 10:1, 8 and Mark 6:7). Later in His ministry He empowered seventy disciples in a similar way, "And heal the sick that are there, and say unto them, The kingdom of God is come near unto you" (Luke 10:9).

During Jesus' last discourse with His apostles, He indicated that because He would go away and the Spirit would be sent, His followers would do greater works than He had done, "He that believeth on me, the works that I do shall he do also; and greater works than these shall he do, because I go unto my Father" (John 14:12). For a discussion showing that this passage speaks of the individual, not the cumulative work of the Church, see Chapter 6.

At His ascension He specifically mentions healing gifts as those being imparted to His followers, "And these signs shall follow those who believe; In my name shall they cast out demons; they shall speak with new tongues; They shall take up serpents;

and if they drink any deadly thing, it shall not hurt them; they shall lay hands on the sick, and they shall recover" (Mark 16:17-18).

Occasionally, someone will say that this commission was for the apostles only, or only for the early church. Jesus specifically says that the signs will follow "those who believe," thus making clear that this would be true for all believers.

The New Testament gives many examples of individuals other than the apostles who operated in these signs. The deacon Stephen "did great wonders and miracles among the people" (Acts 6:8). Acts 8:6-7 mentions the "miracles which he [the deacon and evangelist Philip] did; For unclean spirits, crying with a loud voice, came out of many that were possessed with them; and many taken with palsies, and that were lame, were healed." Ananias, a disciple with no particular office in the church, was used to restore the sight of Saul of Tarsus (Acts 9:10-18). Paul obviously expects the believers in the church in Corinth to be operating in these signs (1 Corinthians 12). Furthermore, as we will note several times, James (chapter 4) exhorts believers to have the elders pray for them, anointing with oil, for healing from illness. Thus, elders are to be operating in this area, at the very least.

The key phrase is "in my name." The use of this phrase indicates that it is not anything in the believers' lives that will produce healing. It will be due to His name, that is, the character of God. Thus, we come full circle and can see that healing itself is based on the character of God Himself.

Since God provided healing in the atonement for all believers (see Chapter 2) and since the character of God involves healing, we are paupers indeed if we do not avail ourselves of His great provision of healing.

[1] See, for example, in Catherine Marshall, *Something More* (Grand Rapids: Chosen Books, 1974), pp.164-167.

2
Basis for Healing in the Atonement

There are many passages in the Bible that deal with healing, and there are many that teach that there is healing available through the atonement of Jesus on the cross. It is essential to understand this doctrine. We will look at some of these passages.

The premier passage is Isaiah 53:

> ¹Who hath believed our report? and to whom is the arm of the LORD revealed? ²For he shall grow up before him as a tender plant, and as a root out of a dry ground: he hath no form nor comeliness; and when we shall see him, *there is* no beauty that we should desire him. ³He is despised and rejected of men; a man of sorrows, and acquainted with grief: and we hid as it were *our* faces from him; he was despised, and we esteemed him not.
> ⁴Surely he hath borne our griefs, and carried our sorrows: yet we did esteem him stricken, smitten of God, and afflicted. ⁵But he *was* wounded for our transgressions, *he was* bruised for our iniquities: the chastisement of our peace *was* upon him; and with his stripes we are healed. ⁶All we like sheep have gone astray; we have turned every one to his own way; and the LORD hath laid on him the iniquity of us all. ⁷He was oppressed, and he was afflicted, yet he opened not his mouth: he is brought as a lamb to the slaughter, and as a sheep before her shearers is dumb, so he openeth not his mouth. ⁸He was taken from prison and from judgment: and who shall declare his generation? for he was cut off out of the land of the living: for the transgression of my people was he stricken. ⁹And he made his grave with the wicked, and with the rich in his

death; because he had done no violence, neither *was any* deceit in his mouth.

[10]Yet it pleased the LORD to bruise him; he hath put *him* to grief: when thou shalt make his soul an offering for sin, he shall see *his* seed, he shall prolong *his* days, and the pleasure of the LORD shall prosper in his hand. [11]He shall see of the travail of his soul, *and* shall be satisfied: by his knowledge shall my righteous servant justify many; for he shall bear their iniquities. [12]Therefore will I divide him *a portion* with the great, and he shall divide the spoil with the strong; because he hath poured out his soul unto death: and he was numbered with the transgressors; and he bare the sin of many, and made intercession for the transgressors.

As we mentioned in the introduction, very few churches in the evangelical mainstream in the United States today teach healing. The only part of this passage from Isaiah that we have ever heard anyone address in connection with healing in these churches is the clause in verse 5: "with his stripes we are healed." We have heard teaching on that clause and the New Testament passage that quotes it, 1 Peter 2:24. These churches use various ways of "explaining away" this phrase. Churches that accept that healing is for the church today tend to quote the phrase without much enlightenment. Churches that teach that healing is not for the church today tend to explain it away by saying something like, "That verse means that in eternity, when we get our resurrection bodies, we will have complete healing. Healing is not available in these mortal bodies. We receive a spiritual healing in this life." The other New Testament passage that quotes from the Isaiah passage, Matthew 8:17, "Himself took our infirmities, and bare our sicknesses" was never mentioned.

As we began to study the Isaiah passage in the original Hebrew, we were astonished at what we discovered. Understanding verses 4-5 and 10-12 is key to understanding that healing is in the atonement.

The word translated "grief" in verses 3 and 4 is חֳלִי, or *choliy*. This word is used twenty-four times in the Old Testament. Twelve times it is translated "sickness"; seven times, "disease"; four times (including the two in this passage), "grief"; and one time, "sick." It comes from a primitive root, חָלָה, or *chalah*, which means "to become sick" or "be diseased or weak". Obviously, the word normally is related to illness or disease.

The word translated "grief" in verse 10 is that primitive root, *chalah*. It is used 75 times in the Old Testament. It is translated "sick" 34 times, and most of the other translations indicate sickness or infirmity. In this verse the *hiphil* stem is used. This stem is causal; in this case it means that God *caused* Jesus to become sick. Looking at the context in that verse ("... he hath put *him* to grief: when thou shalt make his soul an offering for sin..."), we see that Isaiah seems to be saying that God was going to cause Jesus to become sick when he made his soul an offering for sin, another indication that the atonement does in fact include healing.

There were other enlightening words. The word translated "sorrow(s)" in verses 3 and 4, is a word that carries the idea of pain as well as sorrow. "Carried" is just to "carry a load" or to "tote." Thus, by linking pain and sickness twice (in both verse 3 and 4), Isaiah is definitely showing that these sufferings were included in Jesus' sacrifice on the cross.

As we continued our study of this passage, we looked at the word translated "borne" and "bare" in verses 4 and 12. It is the same word in the two verses, נָשָׂא, or *nasa'*, and is the same word as the one used in Leviticus 16:22 to describe the scapegoat, who bore and carried away the sin, "And the goat shall bear upon him all their iniquities unto a land not inhabited: and he shall let go the goat in the wilderness." ***It is used for atonement.***

Thus, this passage in Isaiah uses the same word for Christ's bearing our sicknesses and bearing our sin; furthermore, it is the same word as that used for the scapegoat bearing away the sin of the nation. It goes against all rules of grammar or linguistic interpretation to have the word figurative in one sentence and literal in another unless the passage specifically states that fact.

Thus, when we realized that the same word is used for the sacrificial scapegoat and for Jesus' bearing our sins and for bearing our illnesses, we had to see the truth: *Jesus bore our illnesses.* I like to use salvation as a "fix" on interpreting this passage. In the same manner in which we received salvation (sins already borne or paid for, but we have to appropriate by faith), just so (appropriation by faith) are we to receive health (disease already borne). If we reflect on it all, we can understand the connection. Just as by sin, death (and disease) came upon the human race, so by the atonement, sin and disease have been carried away.

Once we understand the truth of this passage from Isaiah, other Scriptures begin to open in a new way. For example, we can look at the passage in which Matthew quotes a portion of this chapter, Matthew 8:17. All Bible-believing Christians say that Matthew is part of the Holy Spirit-inspired canon of Scriptures. Matthew says, "Himself took our infirmities, and bare our sicknesses." This makes it very plain that Matthew understood Isaiah 53 to include our sicknesses and infirmities in the atonement. **If we say that Isaiah 53 does not teach that sicknesses and infirmities were included in the atonement, then we are saying that Matthew was wrong. If we say this, we say that the Holy Spirit made a mistake, and we are indeed in heresy.**

As mentioned above, Peter quotes from Isaiah 53:5, linking it to the atonement: "Who his own self bore our sins in his own body on the tree, that we, being dead to sins, should live unto righteousness; by whose stripes ye were healed"(1 Peter 2:24). Since the only time that Jesus received stripes was in His sufferings related to His crucifixion, then we must assume that these stripes by which we are healed are part of the atonement.

Some very liberal theologians try to claim that Isaiah 53 does not point to Jesus. Many passages in the New Testament refute this assertion. Jesus Himself makes the claim that Isaiah 53 is about Him: "For I say unto you that this that is written must yet be accomplished in me, And he was reckoned among the transgressors; for the things concerning me have a fulfillment" (Luke 22:37). The last part of Jesus' statement is a direct quote from Isaiah 53:12; thus, Jesus was saying that this part of Isaiah 53:12 would be fulfilled in Him. Matthew (Matthew 8:17) and Peter (1 Peter 2:24 [discussed above]) also claim that Jesus is the subject of Isaiah 53. Philip tells the Ethiopian eunuch that Jesus is the subject of Isaiah 53: "Then Philip opened his mouth, and began at the same scripture [Isaiah 53:7-8], and preached unto him Jesus" (Acts 8:35). Thus, this argument does not stand. What must be done is to interpret Isaiah 53 correctly.

Another very strong argument for healing in the atonement involves a study of healing in the Old Testament. Passages such as Leviticus 14 and 15 will show that healing was often associated with sacrifice. A healed leper had to present a blood sacrifice; in fact, the word *atonement* is used, "…and the priest shall make an atonement for him before the Lord" (Leviticus 14:18). The Old Testament is filled with types that are fulfilled in Christ. Thus, the sin offering is a picture of Jesus' sacrifice on Calvary for our sins. Similarly, the blood sacrifice associated with healing is a picture of Jesus' bearing our sicknesses on Calvary. *We cannot accept one as a picture of Christ and deny the other.* There are many,

many times in the Scriptures when salvation from sin and healing from disease are paired. Some examples follow.

David links them very closely in Psalm 103:1-5: "Bless the LORD, O my soul: and all that is within me, *bless* his holy name. Bless the LORD, O my soul, and forget not all his benefits: **Who forgiveth all thine iniquities; who healeth all thy diseases**; Who redeemeth thy life from destruction; who crowneth thee with lovingkindness and tender mercies; Who satisfieth thy mouth with good *things; so that* thy youth is renewed like the eagle's" [bold face ours].

Jesus links these in one discourse in which He quotes from several passages in Isaiah, including Isaiah 6:20. He said that the eyes and ears of the unbelievers who had heard Him but rejected Him had been closed and dulled "lest at any time they should see with their eyes, and hear with their ears, and should understand with their heart, **and should be converted, and I should heal them**" (Matthew 13:15—bold face ours).

James says, "And the prayer of faith shall save the sick, and the Lord shall raise him up; and if he have committed sins, they shall be forgiven him. Confess your faults one to another, and pray one for another, that ye may be healed…" (James 5:15-16). Although we will discuss this passage in more detail in Chapter 6, we will just note here that James is linking healing and forgiveness of sins.

Thus, we have seen that over and over the Bible shows that Jesus did provide healing in the atonement.

In summary, it would be hard to improve on the statement made by Finis Jennings Dake concerning Christ's atonement:

Mr. S. Weir Mitchell, one of the greatest physicians that has ever lived, said, "Back of each disease there is a cause that no drug can reach." Drugs may deaden pain, kill germs, and counteract certain poisons in the body, but they cannot heal. Many times they harm the body worse than the germs. All healing is done by nature and by God. Drugs may be used as antidotes, but this is the extent of their power. Christ atoned on the cross for sin and for sickness, and God is as willing to heal as He is to forgive of sins. If Christ came to take away sin, He certainly came to take away also sickness, the fruit of sin. The only hindrance in getting the full benefits of Calvary is unbelief and lack of appropriation of the blessings which Christ died to give to all men (Isa. 53:4-5; Matt. 6:16-17; 1 Pet. 2:24; Jas. 5:14-16). God's method is to get rid of the cause of disease, sin, while man's method is to cover up sin and deal with the outgrowth of it. If man would obey God and correct the source, there would be no outgrowth of sin.[1]

I especially like the quote from Dr. Mitchell, "Back of each disease there is a cause that no drug can reach." May we each learn to appropriate all that God has provided in Christ's atonement—healing included.

[1]Finis Jennings Dake, *God's Plan for Man* (Lawrenceville, Georgia: Dake Bible Sales, 1949,1977), p. 241.

Section II

3
What Is Divine Healing?

Having seen that healing was provided in the atonement for every believer, we first need to define divine healing; then we must learn how to appropriate that healing individually. In order to do this, we will examine what we call the "faith principle."

At one level any healing is divine healing. We know that God has absolute control over all events in our lives and in the lives of all men. Thus, when He allows medicine, for example, to make us "well," it is a divine healing in that it would not have happened without His causing it to happen.

We usually mean something else by divine healing, however. Usually we refer to a person's healing of an illness for which there is no "natural" explanation. We usually mean that there was no medicine involved that could "explain" the healing. An example would be that of our friend Sally's healing from cancer, related in Chapters 6 and 9. Normally, when cancer is in the bone, the liver, and the brain, the person is terminally ill. Sally was healed by prayer and the anointing with oil. We call that divine healing, because we see nothing that caused the healing; *i.e.*, God did it. Therefore, it is divine.

For the reasons given above, though, we do not like this terminology, as all healing is from God. John 10:10 states very clearly that Satan does not come *ever* except to steal, kill, or destroy. We have seen that part of God's character revealed in His name *Yhwh rapha* is the eternal healer. Thus, all healing is from God. Nevertheless, we will use the terminology "divine healing" to indicate those times in which no physical tool can be identified for healing.

These areas overlap a lot. When Hezekiah was sick unto death, he asked the Lord to heal him. God answered through the prophet Isaiah that he would add 15 years to his life. Isaiah said: "Take a lump of figs. And they took and laid it on the boil, and he recovered" (2 Kings 20:7). But God had said to Isaiah: "Turn again, and tell Hezekiah…I have heard thy prayer, I have seen thy tears: behold, **I will heal thee**…" (2 Kings 20:5—our emphasis). God says that He healed Hezekiah, but a lump of figs was put on the boil. Thus, the use of "medicine" did not change the fact that it was God Who had healed Hezekiah.

One important note needs to be made. Whenever a person believes that he has been healed, it needs to be verified by medical personnel. This is consistent with the Scriptures. When Jesus healed the lepers, He instructed that they show themselves to the priests for verification and the ritual cleansing (Luke 17:14). Bruce relates in Chapter 7 the sad story of a patient who thought she had received divine healing, who discontinued her medications, and who had to have an amputation as a result. **Thus, healing should always be accompanied by verification and direction of medical personnel.**

4
Understanding the Faith Principle

Now that we have a working definition of divine healing, we can learn how to apply this to a particular individual. In order to do this, we must examine what we call the "faith principle." The opposite of faith is doubt, and we will see that Satan almost always tries to attack the exercise of faith. This is true for salvation as well as for healing. Thus, we must learn how to stand against a counterattack of the healing.

The Role of Faith in the Christian Life

First, we must establish the role of faith in the Christian life. It may seem like a trite expression and one that has been used by scores of preachers and Bible teachers, but the phrase, "Faith is the currency in the Kingdom," is a very true statement. There are two key areas in the Bible that illustrate the principles. Hebrews 11 is the premier chapter in the Bible on faith. We will examine some of it in this chapter. Secondly, many New Testament writers hold up the life of Abraham as the living example of faith principles. Since many books have been written on Abraham and faith principles (see, for example Henry Blackaby's book *Created to be God's Friend* for an excellent study in this area), we will highlight only a few of them.

Hebrews 11:1 gives the classic definition of faith: "Now faith is the substance of things hoped for, the evidence of things not seen." The two key words are *substance* and *evidence*. Although the object of faith is not seen, the evidence is there just as if it were seen. Therefore, faith can be described as substance. It is not something spiritual that cannot be considered to be in the real world. It actually becomes more real that the seen world around a person. The question that naturally follows from this definition is how a person comes to the point of having that faith for healing. We will attempt to show the progression to that point.

The author of Hebrews makes one other critical point. He points out that "…without faith *it is* impossible to please *him*: for he that cometh to God must believe that he is, and *that* he is a rewarder of them that diligently seek him" (Hebrews 11:6). This passage shows that we must have faith in our lives, if we are to please God. Therefore, we see that we must have that faith for healing. Understanding that, we can learn how to obtain it.

Before seeing how to obtain the faith for healing, we will look at some of the people mentioned in Hebrews 11 to see how the faith principle worked out in their lives.

Abel's faith enabled him to give a saving sacrifice: "By faith Abel offered unto God a more excellent sacrifice than Cain, by which he obtained witness that he was righteous, God testifying of his gifts: and by it he being dead yet speaketh" (v. 4). By acting on his faith, Abel effected his salvation.

Enoch actually defeated death because of his faith: "By faith Enoch was translated that he should not see death; and was not found, because God had translated him: for before his translation he had this testimony, that he pleased God" (v. 5). A casual reading of this verse might lead one to think that God translated Enoch apart from any activity on Enoch's part. The language ("by faith Enoch"), however, indicates that it was Enoch's activating faith that allowed God to act by translating Enoch.

Noah saved his household and condemned the world because he exercised his faith: "By faith Noah, being warned of God of things not seen as yet, moved with fear, prepared an ark to the saving of his house; by the which he condemned the world, and became heir of the righteousness which is by faith" (v. 7). It is important to notice that Noah was warned by God about "things not seen as yet." This referred to the fact that there had not been rain on the earth before the flood. Thus, Noah had to believe the Word of the Lord in a matter that he could not test from previous experience. This relates to our discussion of Hebrews 11:1 above in which we noted that faith is the "evidence of things not seen." Rain, heretofore unseen to Noah, had to be more real to Noah than the world as it was at that time. *This principle cannot be overstated: our faith causes the unseen world of faith to be more real than the world around us.*

Verses 8-19 recount the faith of Abraham. As noted above, we suggest reading one of the good books about the faith of Abraham, as he is the model most frequently held up in the Scriptures for faith. Although entire books deal with the faith of Abraham, in passing, we will note a few of the statements in these verses.

Abraham in faith went out from his homeland to another place, not knowing where he was going and dwelling in tents (temporary homes [vs. 8-9]). His faith was that the promises of God (*e.g.*, a country for Abraham) were more real than the external circumstances (tents, strange country). He looked for a city built and made by God (v. 10). His wife Sarah by faith received strength to conceive a child at age ninety (v. 11). The key to her faith was that "she judged him faithful who had promised" (v. 11b). The writer of Hebrews says in verse 12 that "therefore" the seed of Abraham became as the sand of the sea and the stars of the sky in number. In other words, because of that faith, the result was obtained. The implication is that, without faith, the result would not have come. Thus, we see that it is imperative to activate the faith. We will discuss this process in more detail in the next section.

Verses 14-16 explain another key part of the process. The writer says that Abraham, Isaac, and Jacob focused on the country God had promised them. He adds that, if they had focused on the country from which they came (the natural circumstances before God speaks into a situation), they might have returned. Thus, faith must be activated; and we must press on, concentrating on the promises of God and not present circumstances.

Finally, Abraham passed the "big test." God asked him to sacrifice Isaac, the son through whom God had promised the blessing. The writer of Hebrews said that Abraham, by faith, offered him up, thinking that God could raise him from the dead. Here we see a similar principle operating as with Noah. Just as Noah had not seen rain, presumably Abraham had never seen a dead person return to life. He did, however, believe that the promises of God (God had revealed raising the dead to him in a figure [v.19]), though unseen, were more real than his previous experiences.

These few examples are not exhaustive, but they do show that when a person activates his faith and believes the promises of God to be more real than his circumstances or experiences, God somehow is able to work in the situation.

How to Activate Faith: Hearing a *Rhema*

Since faith is necessary in every aspect of life, we need to study what the Bible teaches about activating it. We will see that God's standards do not change. Christians have a limited understanding, at least, of faith as it operates in salvation. We will examine that area and then make application to the area of healing.

Paul gives perhaps the best description of how faith is activated: "So then faith *cometh* by hearing, and hearing by the word of God" (Romans 10:17). The key word in this passage is *word*. There are two Greek words that can mean *word*. These must be understood before we can understand fully the passage from Romans.

One is *logos* (λόγος). A Greek philosopher named Heraclitus first used the term *Logos* around 600 B.C. to designate the divine reason or plan which coordinates a changing universe. Thus, when John calls Jesus the *logos* in John 1, he is indicating that He is the reason or plan that is coordinating the universe. This is similar to what Paul says in Colossians 1: 15-17: "Who is the image of the invisible God, the firstborn of every creature: [16]For by him were all things created, that are in heaven, and that are in earth, visible and invisible, whether *they be* thrones, or dominions, or principalities, or powers: all things were created by him, and for him: [17]And he is before all things, and by him all things consist."

The word *logos* came to be associated with the concept of "word." This meaning of "word" is that which embodies a conception or idea. It can also involve what someone has said, either as a single saying or as a body of sayings. By extension, then *logos* can mean "word," "the sayings of God," the "moral precepts given by God," Old Testament prophecy, a thought, a doctrine, a teaching, a narration, or a "thing spoken of." Thus, the Bible is the Word of God, and Jesus is the Living Word of God (the full expression of God).

The second word that means "word" is *rhema* (ῥῆμα). This word has the connotation of that which has been uttered (an utterance), what one has said, a saying, or a message. The ultimate root of *rhema* is *rheo* (ῥέω), which means "to pour forth" or "to flow." Thus, the meaning of *rhema* is much more fluid than that of *logos*. It looks at *word* as an utterance that is "living and moving." It has a direction to it.

The relationship between the two words where the Bible is concerned is complex. Obviously, there are some overlapping areas with the two words. In general, however, we can say that the Word of God (*logos*), the Bible, is a collective teaching; it is the sayings of God, the thoughts of God, the things He has spoken.

The *rhema*, by contrast, is an utterance of God that reaches a particular person. It is specific and directional; and it flows into a person's life. Many people have experienced a time of reading the Bible, perhaps a passage that has been read many times in the past, when that passage will seem just to "jump out" and catch the person's attention. This is *rhema* in action. It is as though God is uttering that passage at that moment in time just for that individual. It can also refer to the "still, small voice" of God, to an inner "knowing," or to the audible voice of God.

When we look at the passage quoted above from Romans 10:17, "So then faith *cometh* by hearing, and hearing by the word of God," we notice that *word* in this instance is *rhema*. Thus, Paul is saying to have faith, one must first hear the *rhema* of God. That is, one must have a specific utterance directed to him from God. That word, then, gives the person the faith to believe.

For example, Section I of this book would give someone the *logos*, or teaching from God, that healing is in the atonement. One must then have that word, or *rhema*, from God that healing is for him in a particular situation in order to have the faith to believe for the healing. There are scores and scores of Scriptures that speak about healing. God can use any of them to give an individual a *rhema* for healing. He can also speak (*rhema*) through a prophet or through His voice to the individual.

Most Christians instinctively accept this relationship between *logos* and *rhema* in the area of salvation. For example, if one is witnessing to an unbeliever, he gives him *logos*. This comes in the form of Scriptures that explain the facts that man fell into sin; that God provided Jesus as the God-man Who lived a perfect life, died as a substitute for our punishment, rose from the dead, and ascended into heaven; and that salvation is a free gift to a person who exercises faith to believe these things. He normally will cite Scriptures that show these facts. These Scriptures and statements are *logos* to the individual receiving them. At some point one of the parts of this *logos* will "make sense," and "a light bulb will come on" for the person. At that point the person will have the faith to believe and become "saved." This point of the "light bulb" is when the *logos* is activated into a *rhema* for the individual.

Sometimes a person does not receive the *logos* from another individual, but he reads the Bible for himself. There have been many occasions when someone has been reading the Bible, and suddenly something "clicks" and he has faith to believe for salvation. This "clicking" is when the *logos* became a *rhema* for him.

More rarely there have been accounts of people who have lived remotely from any Biblical revelation (as in very remote areas of the world) who have "known" that there is a God like Yahweh, but they have never had anyone explain how to know Him. This is closely related to God Himself speaking to an individual.

We have seen these types of circumstances in action so many times that we frequently do not analyze the process. These three ways of receiving a *rhema* for salvation are similar to the process necessary for a person to receive a *rhema* for his healing. Thus, some people receive a *rhema* when they hear the Word taught. Some people receive a *rhema* when they are reading the Scriptures and when one particular Scripture "jumps out" at them. Others receive a direct Word from God for their healing.

We will note how some individuals have heard "their" *rhema* for healing. Many people get their *rhema* when they are meditating on the *logos*, the written Word. Perhaps this is the most frequent way for this to happen.

Derek Prince, for example, had an incurable skin condition when he was in the army for Great Britain during World War II. When he read Proverbs 4:20-22, he noted that the word translated *health* literally means "medicine": "²⁰My son, attend to my words; incline thine ear unto my sayings. ²¹Let them not depart from thine eyes; keep them in the midst of thine heart. ²²For they *are* life unto those that find them, and health to all their flesh." That last phrase became a *rhema* for him. He tells his story:

> ...[O]ne day the Holy Spirit directed me to Proverbs 4:20-22. This is the passage that got me out of hospital. I want to emphasize the importance of being directed by the Holy Spirit. He is the One who directs us to that particular portion of the Word which represents what we need at any given moment. [This is his way of talking about getting a *rhema*—author's note.]
>
> ...When I got to those last words, "health to all their flesh," I said to myself, "That settles it! Not even a philosopher can make 'flesh' mean 'spirit.'" Flesh is flesh—it is my physical body—and God says He has provided health for all my physical body.
>
> ...So I saw that God had provided "medicine," which He guaranteed would give me health in my whole physical body. I determined to take God's Word as my medicine.
>
> ...So I took God's Word faithfully as my medicine, three times daily after meals, for about three or four months. As a result, I received a complete and permanent

healing. I have walked in that health for nearly forty years from that day until now.[2]

Once he had received his *rhema* for healing, he could stand in absolute faith for his complete healing.

Some people get a *rhema* from a spoken word from God, not from the written word becoming a *rhema*. Bruce received his *rhema* for healing of his rheumatoid arthritis from a word of prophecy given in a meeting. At the time he was not seeking healing directly. He tells his story in more detail in Chapter 7.

Another way that some people get a *rhema* for healing is to receive a direct word from God. This word may come in the form of an audible voice, an internal audible voice, an internal silent voice, or an inner "knowing." I have experienced some of these.

When we were in the middle of a move, I was having some dysrhythmia in my heart. I was feeling horrible, but I felt that God was going to heal me. A physician friend called during that time while Bruce was at the location from which we were moving doing some final work. This friend got very worried and insisted that I go to the hospital. I did not agree, and the conversation ended. He called Bruce and told him that I had agreed to go (he thought that I had). So Bruce came to pick me up to take me to the hospital. I had a kind of image of myself if I went to the hospital. I saw myself "hooked up" to a lot of tubes and placed on lots of medication. I felt very oppressed by the whole scene. When Bruce arrived, I had not had a regular heartbeat in a couple of days. All at once, I "knew" that I could tell Bruce that if my heartbeat were not regular, he could take me to the hospital and that it would be regular. There was no audible or silent word from God; I just *knew* that I could stand up and say, "Feel my pulse," and it would be normal. And it was. That knowing is a *rhema* that allowed me to stand in faith for my healing.

On another occasion, we had journeyed to Florida for some meetings (Bruce details more of these meetings in Chapter 7). I had been suffering from increasing pain and immobility from osteoarthritis. My cervical spine was affected from C4-C7 (the four lower cervical vertebrae). I had severe stenosis and spondylosis. As a result the pain went from the spine area out to the left shoulder area. Frequently the pain ran down the left arm, making it and the left hand numb. I also had fierce headaches as a result. My lumbar spine was also involved. I had severe arthritis in the four lower lumbar spine vertebrae, in the sacrum, and in the sacroiliac joints. I could not stand for any length of time at all and frequently could barely walk. Bruce felt that the degeneration of these bones would cause me to be fairly immobile in the months to come.

We had been to The Mayo Clinic. One doctor looked at my x-rays and said, "Your back is gone." Another doctor stated that my bones looked as if some dog had gnawed big hunks out of them. This was my condition when the prophetic presbytery (referred to in Chapter 7 in Bruce's story) spoke to us.

At the same time the prophetic presbytery spoke healing for Bruce, it also had some words for me. One of the individuals (who had never seen me before) said, "I see in the morning times sometimes there is a real—like a weight—that hangs upon you. The Lord says, 'Daughter, you are going to spring out of the bed, and you are going to pursue the day with new health, and new vigor, and new zeal.'"

What I had not voiced, even to Bruce, was the method I had to use to get out of bed in the mornings. I would push, as if against a heavy weight, until I was in a sitting position. Then I would push again to get my legs over the side of the bed. Then, very slowly and with great difficulty, I would place my feet on the floor and move off the bed. After receiving this word, I did not think too much more about it at the time.

The next morning when the alarm clock went off, I sprang out of bed. A minute or two later, I realized what had happened. I had been healed. It was instantaneous. Though Satan has tried to attack me in these areas and although I have back pains if I do heavy work which would tire anyone (as in moving), I do not have the debilitating pains that I once did. I have not had any pain medication, muscle relaxant, or anti-inflammatory medication (all of which I used at one time) since that time.

When Satan later tried to convince me that I was not healed, I could battle in faith, because that faith had come as a result of the Lord speaking a *rhema* directly to me. Although, in one sense, this healing was announced by a prophet, I did not receive my *rhema* until the next morning when I jumped out of bed. At that point, the spoken word contributed to the inner knowing that I was healed. Then I had the *rhema* and the faith to withstand the subsequent attacks.

Once a person receives a *rhema*, then the choice is his. He can choose to activate his faith and to believe the promise of God instead of looking at the present circumstances.

Plan for a Counterattack

Satan will try to attack a person's healing. This is a major problem, and every person seeking healing needs a full understanding of it. We have noted before that he does not come except to steal, kill, and destroy (John 10:10). If he can create doubt, then the conditions for the healing are not present, and the healing can be lost. This should not be surprising, since entertaining doubt causes a person to deny his *rhema*, in effect. Although initially Satan appears not to be able to inflict the illness again, he can imitate the symptoms. Many people at this point lose faith. This works a little like the situation in which Peter was walking on the water. As long as he kept his eyes on Jesus, he succeeded; but, when he got his eyes on the waves (and thus entertained doubt), he began to sink (Matt. 14:25-32) Jesus summed up Peter's problem: "O thou of little faith, wherefore didst thou doubt" (vs. 31). Apparently, when we let doubt stand, we give Satan an open door, or the legal right, to inflict us again.

We all have heard evangelists emphasize to new believers that Satan will attack their newly expressed faith, many times as early as the first week after the salvation decision. This same principle works in healings, although the time for the attack seems to be about the sixth week most often.

A South African professor did a study of a group of people healed under the ministry of Derek Prince: "In a meeting in Pretoria, South Africa, a theology professor interviewed people as they came down from the platform, taking names, addresses and details. In following them up for six months, he found that about 75 percent retained their healing. Almost everyone had a test of faith after about six weeks, and it was at that point that some lost their healing. Subsequently he presented his report as a theological paper at the university."[3]

It was at this six-week point that Bruce began to lose his healing from rheumatoid arthritis. Had he understood this principle at that time, he might not have had to battle for another two years for the healing to be more stabilized. (See a full account of his story in Chapter 7.)

It is very important to confess the faith that one has appropriated for healing. Confession-and-faith/mouth-and-heart are linked in many places in the Bible. Paul explains salvation in these terms in Romans 10:8-10: "But what saith it? The word is nigh thee, *even* in thy **mouth**, and in thy **heart**: that is, the word of faith, which we preach; That if thou shalt confess with thy **mouth** the Lord Jesus, and shalt believe in thine **heart** that God hath raised him from the dead, thou shalt be saved. For with the **heart** man believeth unto righteousness; and with the **mouth** confession is made unto salvation" [bold face ours]. Thus faith, in this case faith for salvation, is linked with its being in the heart and mouth. Faith is believed in the heart, and it is confessed by the mouth. This principle holds true for healing as well.

Paul links belief and speaking with the spirit of faith in 2 Corinthians 4:13: "We having the same spirit of faith, according as it is written, I believed, and therefore have I spoken; we also believe, and therefore speak."

Thus, although the principle behind healing is easy to understand, usually there is much battle involved before the end result. Occasionally, when someone is too sick to battle, another person may "stand in the gap" for him; but eventually, as he becomes stronger, he will have to fight his own battle to keep his healing. In Chapter 6 we recount how a friend, Susan, fought her battle as she became stronger in the healing process.

In the case of my healing from osteoarthritis, related above, the Lord was gracious and helped in this battle with the counterattack. Two events occurred shortly after the healing that enabled me to know that I had been healed.

The first one occurred two weeks after the healing. I was making one last trip down the stairs one evening to get a drink of water. My foot missed the fourth stair from the bottom. I fell down the rest of the stairs, landed hard on my face (for a minute I thought I would lose some front teeth—they stayed sore for several days), my forearms, and my legs and knees. I noticed that I had a deep cut on my right knee. We went to the hospital for possible stitches; they used the tape to try to preserve some skin that had already turned gray. I was very sore from the fall, *but the amazing thing is that my back was totally unhurt!* I believe God allowed this accident to happen so that I would know that my arthritis had been healed. If I were not healed, this accident would have put my back "out of commission" for weeks or months.

The next occurrence was about three weeks after the healing. We were in Vermont, where we have a time-share vacation. My mother had joined us. Out of all the possible side trips available, she was interested in taking the cog railway up Mount Washington. So we did that. That was 1½ hours up the mountain and 1¼ hours down, with a "bounce, bounce, bounce" on each cog the whole way. The amazing thing is that neither my back nor neck hurt. Before my healing, I would have been in agony by the time we were down.

These two events sealed in my heart that I had indeed been healed. Thus, when the attacks of Satan came—and they did—I was able to withstand them. God does not have to give us such confirmations, but we were so new in understanding that He did give us these confirmations. The unchanging, ever true Word of God is confirmation enough; but God was gracious to give us the extra help at the time.

[1]*Enhanced Strong's Lexicon*, (Oak Harbor, WA: Logos Research Systems, Inc.) 1995.

[2]Derek Prince, *Pages From My Life's Book* (Fort Lauderdale, FL: Derek Prince Ministries, 1987), pp. 48-52.

[3]*Derek Prince Jubilee 1995 Celebration 50th Year in Ministry* (Charlotte, NC: Derek Prince Ministries, 1995), p. 18.

Section III

5
The Spiritual Gifts of Healing

In Section I we studied the doctrine of healing. After establishing that part of God's very character is being the Great Healer, we looked at the Biblical basis for healing. We saw that the Bible does teach that healing was provided in the atonement.

In Section II we learned what divine healing is, and we examined how an individual could take the doctrine of healing and apply it. We saw what is necessary for healing to be efficacious for the believer, and we saw how to transfer knowledge of healing into actual healing. We also discussed the necessity for opposing a counterattack.

In this section we will see many different ways that individuals have been healed. First, we need to develop more fully the teachings of the Bible concerning those people God uses to accomplish healing. Thus, we will study what the Bible teaches about the gifts(s) of healing. Then we will look at the three broad categories of the ways God heals. Finally, Bruce will recount his healing journey, as it encompasses many of the principles contained in this book.

One important fact needs to be mentioned whenever we refer to the individual(s) God uses when He heals, and that is that it is God Who is doing the healing. When Peter was used to heal Aeneas, he said to him, "Aeneas, **Jesus Christ maketh thee well**; arise, and make thy bed" (Acts 9:34—our emphasis). With that principle in mind we will examine the spiritual gift(s) of healing.

Gifts of the Spirit

There is a lot of confusion in Christian circles concerning gifts of the Spirit in general. Some groups almost totally ignore the gifts bestowed by the Holy Spirit upon the Church. Others tend to call almost any activity a working of spiritual gifts. We need to see what the Bible teaches in this area.

The word usually used in the New Testament for *spiritual gifts* comes from the Greek word χάρισμα, or *charisma*. This word, in turn comes from a root word, χάρις, or *charis*, meaning *grace, favor,* or *thanks*. *Charisma* is a neuter plural word; this form gives it a basic meaning of "the grace things." Thus these "things" are bestowed by the grace of God. We do not choose them; nor can we earn them.

Paul indicates this in Romans 12:6: "Having then gifts differing according to the grace that is given to us...." This is the same word translated *gift* in Romans 6:23: "For the wages of sin *is* death; but the gift of God *is* eternal life through Jesus Christ our Lord." Here Paul is referring to the free, unmerited favor that God confers on us at the point of salvation. We see, therefore, that the basic meaning is that of an unmerited gift from God.

This word is used seventeen times in the New Testament. Three times it refers to the free gift of salvation; twelve times it refers to the gifts of the Spirit; one time it refers possibly to both; and once it refers apparently to a gift sent to Paul. Overwhelmingly, then, most of the times that this word is used are with reference to spiritual gifts. Our purpose is not to do an in-depth study of the spiritual gifts, but some clarification is needed in order to understand the gifts of healing.

There are several places where Paul lists spiritual gifts. One of the most quoted is 1Corinthians 12:4-11:

⁴Now there are diversities of gifts, but the same Spirit. ⁵And there are differences of administrations, but the same Lord. ⁶And there are diversities of operations, but it is the same God which worketh all in all. ⁷But the manifestation of the Spirit is given to every man to profit withal. ⁸For to one is given by the Spirit the word of wisdom; to another the word of knowledge by the same Spirit; ⁹ To another faith by the same Spirit; to another the gifts of healing by the same Spirit; ¹⁰ To another the working of miracles; to another prophecy; to another discerning of spirits; to another *divers* kinds of tongues; to another the interpretation of tongues: ¹¹But all these worketh that one and the selfsame Spirit, dividing to every man severally as he will.

The word *charisma* is used in verses 4 and 9. In verse 4 Paul is simply saying that although the same Spirit (*i.e.*, the Holy Spirit) gives gifts (v. 7), there are diversities of gifts. In this passage he lists nine of these diversities of operations—word of wisdom, word of knowledge, discerning of spirits, faith, gifts of healing, working of miracles, prophecy, tongues, and interpretation of tongues. Some individuals teach that these nine diversities are the only "spiritual gifts," but this fails to take into account other passages of Scripture.

In Romans 12:6-8, for example, Paul mentions gifts differing according to the grace given to us. He lists prophecy, ministry, teaching, exhortation, giving, ruling, and showing mercy. Since the same word is used for *gifts* in verse 6 as in 1 Corinthians 12:4,9, all interpretation models demand that the lists be of the same thing. Thus, both passages list spiritual gifts.

In at least two passages Paul mentions that people who have certain gifts or people who fill a particular office have been placed in certain churches as gifts to those churches. In Ephesians

4:8-13 Paul states that when Jesus ascended to His Father, He gave gifts unto men: "⁸When he ascended up on high, he led captivity captive, and gave gifts unto men....¹¹And he gave some, apostles; and some, prophets; and some, evangelists; and some, pastors and teachers; ¹²For the perfecting of the saints, for the work of the ministry, for the edifying of the body of Christ: ¹³Till we all come in the unity of the faith, and of the knowledge of the Son of God, unto a perfect man, unto the measure of the stature of the fulness of Christ."

The word for gifts in verse 8 is δόμα (*doma*) from δίδωμι (*didomi*). *Didomi* is a word indicating a simple act of giving. *Doma* is used only four times in the Scriptures and always means "gift." There is no especial connotation of unmerited favor as there is with the word *charisma*. Thus, Paul says that Jesus sent gifts to men. These gifts are listed in verse 11; the gifts are obviously the people who are functioning in certain offices. Thus, in this case apostles, prophets, evangelists, pastors, and teachers are not spiritual gifts or unmerited gifts **given** to people; they **are** people in certain positions or offices. They have been given to some [groups, bodies, churches] to function until all believers have come into the unity of the faith, fully in Christ's image.

In another passage Paul again lists positions in the body of Christ: "²⁷Now ye are the body of Christ, and members in particular. ²⁸And God hath set some in the church, first apostles, secondarily prophets, thirdly teachers, after that miracles, then gifts of healings, helps, governments, diversities of tongues. ²⁹*Are* all apostles? *are* all prophets? *are* all teachers? *are* all workers of miracles? ³⁰Have all the gifts of healing? do all speak with tongues? do all interpret? ³¹But covet earnestly the best gifts: and yet shew I unto you a more excellent way" (1 Corinthians 12:27-31).

In this passage he mentions people set in the church—apostles, prophets, teachers, miracles, gifts (*charisma*) of healing, helps, governments, diversities of tongues. It is interesting that gifts of healing, helps, governments, diversities of tongues sound like a list of gifts, but they are listed in the group of people set in the churches. We can conclude that there is a very fine line between gifts and the gifted ones.

Peter tells us what we are to do with our various gifts (this would include healing): "As every man hath received the gift, even so minister the same one to another, as good stewards of the manifold grace of God" (1 Peter 4:10). We should notice in passing that Peter indicates that **every man** (writing to believers) has received the gift (*charisma*).

Paul tells Timothy not to neglect the gift (*charisma*) that is in him, which was given him by a prophetic presbytery (1 Timothy 4:14); he also tells him (2 Timothy 1:6) to stir up his gift (*charisma*).

With all spiritual gifts, there needs to be a word of explanation. Every believer has some measure of all of the gifts, although people who have a particular gift in a heavy portion are said to have that gift. For example, all believers have a measure of faith; all are expected to use that faith in various circumstances in life. Some believers, however, have an extra measure of faith to the point that it is a spiritual gift. All believers can, at various times, receive a word of knowledge; but some believers operate in using this gift to a larger degree.

Similarly, some believers have the gifts of healing; they should be operating in this gift regularly; ***but all believers can be used in a healing***. We have quoted Mark 16:17-18, where we are told that certain signs shall follow those who believe, including laying hands on the sick for recovery. James also indicates the universal nature of operating in healing for believers: "Confess *your* faults one to another, and pray one for another, that ye may be healed. The effectual fervent prayer of a righteous man availeth much" (James 5:16).

The Spiritual Gifts of Healing

Thus, we have seen that there is a gift of the Holy Spirit, called gifts of healing, which is given to some people; they should not neglect that gift; they should stir it up at all times. Since we know that the Holy Spirit has given this gift to certain people and has placed them in various churches, we should be seeing quite a bit of use of this gift today. The fact that we do not see this gift in operation very much is evidence of the poverty of the Church today.

We need to examine one facet of the gifts of healing. In all the lists that mention healing, the gift is called gifts (plural) of healing. We should ask why the gift is always mentioned in the plural.

I believe, but cannot prove, that one reason is that there are two types of gifts of healing. One is the gift of healing given to a believer by the Holy Spirit. This gift, as with all the spiritual gifts, is given by the Holy Spirit, as He pleases (1 Corinthians 12:11).

Then there is that given to those who stand in one of the five offices listed above in Ephesians 4. (We should note that some scholars feel that the original indicates that pastors and teachers are the same office. In this case there would be four offices. The principles we are developing are the same for either interpretation.) If we look at the New Testament, we see that those who had any of the offices listed in Ephesians 4 also operated in healing gifts. (Just as He gives the gifts to believers, so the Holy Spirit also gives the offices to individuals and, in turn, the gifted people to the Church.)

Thus, Philip was an evangelist, and listed with his evangelism are acts of healing: "For unclean spirits, crying with a loud voice, came out of many that were possessed with them; and many taken with palsies, and that were lame, were healed" (Acts 8:7).

Peter, as an apostle, operated in the healing gifts (Acts 3:1-11; 5:15; 9:32-41;). Paul, as an apostle, operated in the healing gifts throughout his ministry (e.g., Acts 19:12). Other apostles also performed many healing miracles (Acts 5:12,16).

Silas is called a prophet (Acts 15:32) and apparently participated with Paul in healings (e.g., Acts 16). Timothy is a pastor and a teacher; Paul alludes to sign gifts, which would include healing, in 2 Timothy 4:5b: "…do the work of an evangelist, make full proof of thy ministry."

Using the Gifts of Healing

Thus, we have seen that some people have the gift of healing, and we have seen that everyone who operates in one of the offices listed in Ephesians 4 should be exercising the gifts of healing. In addition, every believer can pray the prayer of faith, and the sick will recover (James 5:16).

It is not from lack of the Holy Spirit's gifting believers that the gift of healing is not seen operating much today. Rather, it is that God's people have failed to identify their gifts, use their gifts, or even know about spiritual gifts. We need to remind ourselves of the words with which Paul exhorted Timothy: "Neglect not the gift that is in thee, which was given thee by prophecy, with the laying on of the hands of the presbytery....I put thee in remembrance that thou stir up the gift of God..." (1 Timothy 4:14; 2 Timothy 1:6a).

We are told that in the early church people brought the sick on beds in order for them to be healed by the shadow of Peter passing by and that many sick people from the cities around Jerusalem were healed. "And they were healed every one" (Acts 5:16). How far below this level of using our spiritual gifts have we fallen!

We should note parenthetically a factor that should be considered in all healings. It is beyond the scope of this booklet to examine such areas as demon possession or influence, but it is a real source of many illnesses. A look at Jesus' healing ministry will show that frequently the line between pure physical illness and an illness inflicted by Satan is very fine. Many people who have worked in this area stress that it is helpful to have a person present at a healing (whether it be the person who is an instrument of healing or a fellow worker) who has discernment in the spirit as to the cause of the problem. Derek Prince, for example, who has had scores of years dealing in these areas, says: "...not all sicknesses are caused by demons. Many have other, natural causes. This makes it important to identify sicknesses that are directly caused by demons. In 1 Corinthians 12 Paul lists nine supernatural gifts of the Holy Spirit available to believers. Of these there are two that may help us to identify demons: literally, *a word of knowledge* and *discernings of spirits* [*sic*] (see verse 8,10)."[1]

Thus, we must conclude that an essential part of the Church's seeing healing for God's people today is for everyone to play his part. We must identify our spiritual gifts and then use them. In addition, each believer should, when necessary, pray the prayer of faith and be delivered from illness and infirmity. We have been in bondage to Satan entirely too long!

[1]Derek Prince, *They Shall Expel Demons* (Grand Rapids: Chosen Books, 1998), p. 199.

6
Various Methods God Uses to Heal

There are many methods that God uses to heal individuals. Although no two healings are ever totally alike, there are three general categories under which *most* of them fall.

One is **the direct miracle**. This miracle can occur as a direct, sovereign act of God; or God may use an individual to impart the healing. This individual can be any believer who prays for the individual in faith, sometimes accompanied by the laying on of hands; or it can be a believer with the gift of healing.

Another method is healing by **prayer offered on behalf of the ill person**, with or without that person's active participation. The method of laying on of hands and anointing with oil by the elders falls into this category.

Probably the most commonly used method is **the prayer of faith** prayed by the ill individual with or without agreement of other believers. This method may seem to be the most varied, since various individuals come to the point of faith in many different ways, but the method is the same—prayer backed up by faith.

Although we can isolate these three types of healing, in many cases they overlap. Nevertheless, these categories will be examined in more detail.

The Direct Miracle

This category of healing is possibly the least considered in the church today. Many of us have absorbed the humanistic way of thinking about the universe. We tend to think that God created the universe (if we even credit God with creation!), set it into motion, established "laws" by which it could operate, and then left it to run on its own. This is one of Satan's great lies for the post-Reformation world.

The fact is that we live in a supernatural universe, and we live under a God Who wants to intervene in the lives of His children. Since He does not violate our volition, He is limited many times by the fact that we never ask Him to act on our behalf.

This is not the way God wants us to operate. Jesus made this very clear immediately before His ascension. He told the disciples: "And these signs shall follow them that believe; In my name shall they cast out devils; they shall speak with new tongues; They shall take up serpents; and if they drink any deadly thing, it shall not hurt them; they shall lay hands on the sick, and they shall recover" (Mark 16:17-18).

Thus, the **normal** signs that would accompany believers would be casting out demons, speaking with new tongues, immunity from such things as poisonous snakes, and ability to heal. This promise was not made just to the eleven apostles, to the disciples who had seen Jesus, to deacons or to elders, or to any special group of believers. It was given to "them that believe." We should all be operating in these areas. The application for healing, however, is that any believer should be able to lay hands on a sick person and see that person restored if other conditions are met (see Chapter 7).

The word *signs* is σημεῖον (semeion), which has a meaning of "sign, miracle, or mark." It comes from a root word meaning "mark." The idea is that the ability to lay hands on sick people and to have them healed is a *sign* or *mark* of those who believe.

Sometimes the miracle occurs without the laying on of hands. Many times God sovereignly decides to move in a situation. Every time is so different that these occurrences are almost impossible to categorize. This was true of the miracles that Jesus performed during His earthly ministry. Appendix A shows some of the ways Jesus healed. It is not an exhaustive list of those whom Jesus healed, but it serves to show the variety of ways He used.

Lest someone say that those types of healings apply to Jesus only and not the church, Jesus Himself made it very plain that, after He would ascend to the Father, the church would do greater miracles than He had done. He said, "Verily, verily, I say unto you, He that believeth on me, the works that I do shall he do also; and greater *works* than these shall he do; because I go unto my Father. And whatsoever ye shall ask in my name, that will I do, that the Father may be glorified in the Son. If ye shall ask any thing in my name, I will do *it*" (John 14:12-14).

Many people have tried to interpret these verses as applying to the cumulative works of the Church. They say that if we count the works of believers from the time of Christ until now, they constitute a greater amount than those done by our Lord. This interpretation cannot be sustained from the passage. In verse 12, Jesus uses the word *he* three times. This word is masculine singular and is part of the verb. In Greek it is sufficient to use the verb form that includes the word *He* as the subject. In this passage, however, the article *the* in the masculine, singular form is used before one of the verbs in addition to emphasize that Jesus was speaking of a single individual. It simply cannot be used in a collective sense.

In the context of the passage, since Jesus immediately goes on to talk about the fact that His departure will allow the Father to send the Holy Spirit, we can assume that it is the gift of the indwelling Holy Spirit that allows believers during this age to perform that kind of miracles. The Bible is clear that we are to be asking God to heal individuals through direct miracles.

The New Testament record makes it plain that the early church believed this. Nothing in the Scriptures can possibly be interpreted to mean that the miracle of healing was to cease at any time during the Church Age (see discussion in Chapter 8).

Prayer Offered on Behalf of the Ill Individual

Whereas miracles occur only when, where, and how the Sovereign God ordains, every believer can and should avail himself of healing through prayer. The Lord frequently heals when prayer is offered on behalf of the ill individual; and many times the believer will pray for himself, especially when he has obtained a *rhema* for his healing. Prayer offered on behalf of the ill individual normally occurs in one of two ways. Any believer can pray for the ill individual in this way, as we will see below. Another method is that the elders lay hands on the sick individual and anoint with oil. Both of these methods are described in the Scriptures.

Prayer Offered by a Believer for a Sick Individual

The prayer offered by a believer for a sick individual may be with or without his active participation. When the prayer is without his participation, it is normally because the person is so ill that he is unable to participate. This would include an individual in a coma or a person who is so weak that he does not have the strength to participate. In cases in which people are conscious, but weak, they frequently can participate by giving their assent. This method is totally in line with many Scriptures. One is James 5:16: "Confess *your* faults one to another, and pray one for another, that ye may be healed. The effectual fervent prayer of a righteous man availeth much." The passage indicates that we must confess known sin (see Chapters 9 and 10 for more discussion of confession of sin before prayer for healing), and then it commands us to pray for one another. Yes, this is another command; the verb *pray* is imperative, meaning a command.

Mark tells us to *expect* this type of healings: "And [Jesus] said unto them, Go ye into all the world, and preach the gospel to every creature.... And these signs shall follow them that believe... they shall lay hands on the sick, and they shall recover" (16:15-18).

A close personal friend of ours was healed in this manner. Susan wrote her own story. Parts of it are excerpted below with certain identifying features and names changed (all underlined words in the original).

My sister, Annabelle, who stood by me through so many years of illness, was shown in a dream that she and my nephew, Travis, were to agree on the verse Matthew 18:19, "If two shall agree on earth as touching anything that they shall ask, it shall be done for them of my Father which is in Heaven." ...She was shown that they were to believe for my complete healing.

[The previous day] she had come to my house and after one look at me, she told Travis, "If we are ever going to pray in earnest for her healing it had better be now.... she won't be alive much longer." She went home to pray and the Lord gave her the dream.

Travis agreed, as it seems the Lord had been leading him in the same direction. [Travis was a medical student and was spending some time with me during the summer.] It was about that time that my nights were so restless due to the illness....I walked to the front door, having heard a soft summer rain. I was so feverish I wanted to stand on the porch and feel the cool rain. I found Travis standing outside on the porch; and when he turned, there were tears in his eyes and he abruptly said, "You know you are going to die, don't you, and that it will be a violent death in convulsions?" I said, "Yes." He said, "I can't stand to ... leave you like this....if it is all right with you, I am going to pray that God heal you and if not, that He take you quickly." So obviously God was moving both of them to action...this was God's time, and they both knew this as Annabelle shared her dream.

Travis was led to pray for one illness at a time, which they did. They entered into almost constant prayer and fasting, agreeing to fast until the Lord started the healing process. They continued in prayer and in His word for a period of almost two weeks. Many times I would get out of bed and walk down the hall to Travis' room and find him on his knees by the bed with his open Bible before him. They would lay hands on me and pray many times each day....and rebuke the devil, as we are instructed to do in the Word. They claimed promises and used Scripture (our weapon) that Christ gave us to use...always basing their faith on Matt. 18:19. So this was Scriptural and in direct line with the Word of God.

This was a rather large order as I had been quite ill for a number of years...with several organic disorders and diseases. I had pyelitis (urinary tract infection renal insufficiency, uremia [early stages] and hypertension) of both kidneys with proteus present. At that time there were no antibiotics that could control the proteus factor. (Some of the other bacteria could be checked temporarily with antibiotics....) My different urologists had said it was incurable. I had not been without antibiotics for this condition for over two and one-half years. I was under the care of several doctors at all times and spent months in bed and a week to ten days in the hospital many times. The last hospitalization prior to my healing I was hospitalized a full month.

I had a history of ulcers. Medicines and diet did not prevent the recurrence of these ulcers, which threatened to perforate the duodenum on several occasions. The doctors recommended surgery, but my body was not in condition to tolerate another operation due to other infections in my body. I had low blood pressure and was chronically underweight for years.

[She then lists several other, less life-threatening conditions.] My total intake of drugs was thirty-one to forty-three pills each day, depending on the type and amount of antibiotics being prescribed at the time.

At the very onset of their agreeing in prayer I went into a severe kidney attack with chills and high fever and aching and nausea. The kidney problem was the first thing they agreed on...while I was in the midst of the worst attack to date. Once they had started in prayer, I sent all of my pills and medication of every kind to the alley for disposal. We looked to the Lord only!

Perhaps I should add here that the only part I played in this was my faith in God's faithfulness to His Word, and

His Word was the basis for their agreement in prayer. The day they started praying for the ulcers I abandoned my diet of little other than milk at that time, and beginning that day I ate exactly everything that everyone else ate and had no ill effects then or since!

As each disease or disorder was healed, they thanked God and praised Him and agreed on the next item! I was completely healed! I took no medicine and felt wonderful. The digestive tract and intestinal tract functioned perfectly. I gained thirteen pounds in two weeks. I even had corns under two toenails that were quite painful and had been present for years. They dropped out in a day.

I am a living testimony of what God can and will do. I don't claim to have all the answers about healing... no one does, because you can't put God in a mold, and I have not ever seen any two healings alike. I have had many healings in my lifetime, but no two have been the same. How does one express their [sic] awe that God cares so tenderly for His children and hears and answers prayer? How do we comprehend His grace provisions on the Cross for mankind? Even now I am amazed at His gracious provision! There was no merit in me that God should extend His hand of mercy...but thankful? Oh yes, but not ever thankful enough, I know...anymore than we can ever thank Him enough or praise Him enough for our salvation.

Oh yes, another thing I wanted to share! The second week into the healing process when we were all in agreement I began reading the New Testament and Psalms three times each day after meals and at bedtime. As a minister [Note: this is the testimony of Derek Prince, which we discussed in Chapter 4.] brought out one time if you were taking medicine wouldn't it be taken according to those directions? And if God is your source of health (and your "medicine" shall we say) then would not this be the logical way to schedule the intake of The Word as your source of health and strength?

And so each time I would remind the Lord that according to Proverbs 4:20-22, "My son, attend to my words, incline thine ear unto my saying. Let them not depart from thine eyes; keep them in the midst of thine heart, For they are life unto those that find them, and health to all their flesh." And then I would "take in" the Word, at least one chapter and usually many chapters. Even now when I come across [the Bible I used in those days] I find myself holding it a moment in my hands remembering that miraculous time in my life.[1]

Although we are putting Susan's story in this section that discusses the prayer that believers can offer for other people, many of the principles in healing are mentioned in her story. Her sister and nephew were able to pray in faith only after they had a *rhema*. This was in the form of a dream for Annabelle, and it was an inner knowing for Travis. Both agreed on a Scripture for their praying. Although Susan initially was too ill to pray for herself, she makes a point of saying that "the only part I played in this was my faith in God's faithfulness to His Word...." Thus, her agreement and faith were important. After the healing process began and after it concluded, she actively assumed a role in faith. She applied the Scriptures three times a day in faith. Her activated faith, therefore, would help her maintain her healing in spite of counterattacks, and she did have numerous counterattacks. She maintained her healing of these ailments the rest of her life, some thirty-five years. She notes that healing, like salvation, is one of His grace provisions earned on the Cross. She gives full credit to God for the healing, stating that it was a gift of grace; and she acknowledges that healing was provided on the Cross. Her sister, nephew, and she were careful to do two things. As each problem was healed, they thanked God for that. Secondly, they did not admit anyone to their prayers who had any doubt about God's healing (note our discussion of this important principle in Chapter 10). This is in line with instructions from James 1:6-7: "But let him ask in faith, nothing wavering. For he that wavereth is like a wave of the sea driven with the wind and tossed. For let not that man think that he shall receive any thing of the Lord." The testimony of her nephew, who is a doctor, gives a medical verification of the healing.

I used this method of simple prayer for healing with a friend who had terminal cancer. Sally had struggled with cancer for several years. Finally, the cancer was in most of her organs, including her chest, bones, and liver. Her doctor thought she had only a month to live. None of the chemotherapy or radiation had worked. In fact, she was given a treatment called salvage chemotherapy. This is basically given when the doctors determine that none of the known combination of drugs will work, and some experimental doses are put together. I went to stay with her for a few days, expecting to have to say earthly "goodbyes." The first day I was there Sally contracted pneumonia and nearly did not survive through the next twelve hours. When she stabilized from that, her doctor thought that she would not live more than fourteen days. At that point I began anointing her with oil, laying hands on her head and in the liver area, and praying twice a day. The cancer was so progressive that her abdomen area looked like a woman ready to deliver a baby. When I began praying, her nausea abated; and gradually her abdomen began to shrink. Within a month the cancer indicators in her blood were approaching normal. Her HMO did a scan, which showed no trace of cancer. The HMO was so amazed that it ran a second scan (and it is a notoriously stingy HMO and not one that typically runs unnecessary scans).

There was no trace of cancer; in fact, the report stated that the formerly affected areas looked as if there had been surgery in that area. Of course, there had not been (except God's surgery). This scan meets the criterion of having healings documented by medical records when possible.

When I first began the prayer, I had Sally's assent. Sally was too sick to battle actively in prayer. She did believe, however, that God wanted to heal her. In fact, shortly before becoming ill she had received a *rhema* for her healing in a dream. We relate this and the ending of the story in Chapter 9.

Laying on of Hands and Anointing with Oil by the Elders

Any ill believer can and should avail himself of the opportunity of being anointed with oil by the elders of his church at any time. We are told in James 5:14-15: "Is any sick among you? **let him call** for the elders of the church; and let them pray over him, anointing him with oil in the name of the Lord: And the prayer of faith shall save the sick, and the Lord shall raise him up; and if he have committed sins, they shall be forgiven him" [our emphasis]. The words "let him call" are interesting. They are one word, a verb, in Greek. The verb is third person singular (thus, the "him"); it is aorist tense, which indicates a single action. In other words, the action described in these verses needs to be done only once; it is not a "continuing action" verb. In addition, it is in the middle voice. We have only active and passive voices in English. Middle voice indicates that the subject (he) does the acting but that the action results in the subject's being acted upon. (In other words, the person acts—he calls for the elders of the church; but he is acted upon—he is anointed with oil and healed). Most important is the mood of the verb. It is imperative; *that is a command*. We have no choice. The sick person is commanded to call for the elders of the church. **There is no other direct command in the Bible concerning**

illness. How few are the people who do this, and how few are the churches that encourage their members to follow this command! When we know something to be in God's will and do not do it, we have little basis to pray for results in that area. From this passage we know that God's will is for us to call upon the elders of our church. This should be the first step that any ill believer takes. It should be done before seeking medical attention. We understand this by noticing that although there were physicians in the New Testament period, this command was still given.

We have seen remarkable healings from having the elders pray and anoint with oil. Evan, a friend of ours, was diagnosed with acute myeloid leukemia, which is one of the most aggressive forms of the disease. He asked the elders of the church to anoint him with oil and to pray for his healing. The disease went into complete remission for about a year. All medical tests showed him to be cancer-free. This form of leukemia normally does not respond in this way. This must be seen as a healing miracle for Evan. Unfortunately, there were some forces of unbelief operating within his close circle. We believe that this contributed to the eventual return of the disease. We discuss this problem of doubt within the circle of prayer in Chapter 10.

It was the example of this friend that first caused Bruce to examine the passage in James 5 concerning the anointing with oil and prayer by the elders. This led to his rising faith (*rhema*). As a result, he had the faith to ask the elders to pray for his right ankle, which was so painful that he could hardly walk. That pain left within a week of the prayer and has never returned. That has been 15 years at this point. At that point we did not understand much of the Bible's teaching about healing, and we did not understand that Bruce could have and should have asked for prayer for the disease that had crippled his ankle, rheumatoid arthritis. Bruce tells more about this in the next chapter.

The Prayer of Faith Offered by the Ill Individual

Probably the most common prayer for healing is that offered by the ill individual who understands God's plan for healing. There are many Scriptures God has provided for healing by those praying the prayer of faith. In fact, scores of people have claimed many varied Scriptures for healing, with results. We believe that God gives faith to individuals and that their asking God for healing is answered because of the character of God. That is why we spent time in Sections I and II developing the doctrine of healing, the doctrine of the character of God, and the meaning of *rhema* and the place it plays in bringing us to have the faith upon which to stand.

The following steps should be taken by the person who wishes to pray the prayer of faith for healing. First, recognize that faith cannot be somehow "magically" assumed. One must immerse himself in the Scriptures dealing with healing and spend much time in communion with the Lord. The two primary ways of hearing from God are through reading His Word and through communion with Him. Of course, God in His sovereignty and mercy sometimes meets an individual who is not seeking in this fashion, but normally one must seek Him through one of these ways to hear from Him.

Thus, for healing, when we are reading or meditating on Scripture and a word of faith seems to leap out at us, vying for our attention, then God is giving us a *rhema* for our healing. We are to take that word, pray it in faith, confess our healing, and hold fast to it. That is how the prayer of faith works. It is very important, therefore, for us to immerse ourselves with the Scriptures—before we need them for a healing—so that they are hidden in our hearts at the time of need. I believe that reading the Gospel accounts of Jesus' ministry and seeing that He never turned anyone away for healing can cause this faith to rise. It is possible to approach the Lord simply as did the people in Jesus' earthly ministry and ask directly for healing.

There is testimony after testimony of individuals who have been healed using the prayer of faith. By looking at some of them, we can see that many different Scriptures have served as a *rhema* for different people. We believe that it is not the individual Scripture that is important. **As with every area of the Christian life, what God wants is *relationship*.** This concept cannot be overstressed. The fellowship with God, getting to know Him, and abiding in Him are the items of value in our lives. The healing is simply a wonderful side effect.

Many people have had healing on the basis of Matthew 18:19: "Again I say unto you, That if two of you shall agree on earth as touching any thing that they shall ask, it shall be done for them of my Father which is in heaven." This Scripture is used many times when two or three people are agreeing in prayer for a healing. We recounted Susan's healing, using this Scripture, earlier in the chapter.

One of the most commonly used Scriptures when the individual is praying for himself is Mark 11:23-24: "For verily I say unto you, That whosoever shall say unto this mountain, Be thou removed, and be thou cast into the sea; and shall not doubt in his heart, but shall believe that those things which he saith shall come to pass; he shall have whatsoever he saith. Therefore I say unto you, What things soever ye desire, when ye pray, believe that ye receive *them*, and ye shall have *them*." The sequence of tense in the last part of verse 24 is very important. Jesus says, "*When* ye pray, *believe*...." One has to believe that he receives the healing **at the same time he is praying**. Then, the external signs or manifestation of that prayer will follow ("ye *shall* have them"). Many of us pray, then look at our circumstances and see no evidence of a change, and then conclude that we are not healed. Jesus says to pray, believing that we have the petition; He then promises that we will have it at some time in the future. Kenneth Hagin used this verse as a boy of sixteen to be healed of an incurable heart disease and partial paralysis. He lived after his healing nearly 70 years (until the time of his death) in total health.[2]

One Scripture used successfully by many people is Proverbs 4:20-22: "My son, attend to my words; incline thine ear unto my sayings. Let them not depart from thine eyes; keep them in the midst of thine heart. For they *are* life unto those that find them, and health to all their flesh." The word translated "health" is literally medicine. The word translated "flesh" *always* means flesh; it can never have a spiritual meaning. Thus, those people who say that healing in this life is really just spiritual and that we cannot have physical healing in this life have serious trouble with this verse. We saw in Chapter 4 that this was the verse claimed by Derek Prince in the deserts of North Africa in World War II for a skin disease incurable at that time in that place. He realized that most people take medicine three times a day and thus "took" the Word three times a day for healing. We also noted earlier in this chapter that Susan used the same Scripture as she became well enough to pray the prayer of faith for herself.

Scriptures that show that God wants us healed or that healing is associated with salvation are effective. See Psalm 103:1-5, Exodus 15:26, Matthew 8:3, Matthew 9:2-8, Matthew 13:15, and 3 John 2. There are, of course, many more. There are so many Scriptures that people have used in praying the prayer of faith that we could not develop the use of all of them. The most helpful tool for this is a complete concordance of the Bible. A person should take the concordance and note every verse in the Bible that concerns healing. One man did this, marking each passage on healing in his Bible in blue. He notes that his Bible looked like the ocean! There are many computer programs that will print every verse containing a certain word. A person could print these and begin to meditate on them.

In this rather lengthy chapter we have seen that there are three large categories of methods God used to heal—the direct miracle, prayer offered on behalf of the ill individual, and the prayer of faith prayed by the ill individual. Since every healing is very personalized by God, these categories are simply general guides. God wants to heal us even more than we want to be healed, but He does want a relationship with us more. As we focus on our relationship with Him, healing will become as natural to us as any other kind of prayer.

[1] Personal letter to the author

[2] Kenneth Hagin relates his healing story in many of his booklets—*e.g.*, *I Believe in Visions* (Tulsa: Faith Library Publications, 1993), pp. 24-27.

7
Bruce's Journey of Healing

Note: This chapter is Bruce's story in his own words.

1. Introduction

I am including my narrative in this book about healing, since it illustrates many of the points that are made in the text. One of the major reasons for writing this book was to fill a need that we found when searching for truth related to God's healing us. We hope that our story will help other people to understand more about divine healing. God is always rational, kind, and merciful. If we seek Him for information, He will answer us. Much of our information has been obtained in answered prayer.

Divine healing is an extremely difficult subject with which to grapple, for many reasons. For example, I believe that God supernaturally healed me of rheumatoid arthritis in 1995. When this occurred, I was very surprised; and the healing left me with many questions. Among the more troubling questions were why God chose to heal me and how this healing impacted me as a medical practitioner. Other people might have similar questions when faced with divine healing, but some would have other questions as well.

First, we must have a definition of divine healing so that we can understand what it is and what it is not. From a study of physiology and pathology one learns that there is an ordered progression in the resolution of any illness. For example, there is a basic pathology that can be studied involving the "acute in-flammatory response." This process goes into action when the body experiences an injury from a chemical, infectious agent, or trauma. It runs a course over a period of days. There are some well-known factors that can lengthen or shorten it. This process is something that God gave to us as a mercy, for it helps bring healing to all of His created people whether they have accepted His salvation or not.

A divine healing is a healing that clearly goes outside the statistical norms of a natural process. For example, when I was healed of rheumatoid arthritis (I recount the complete story later in this chapter), I was vastly improved within two days without the use of any additional medications. A natural remission would not have occurred as rapidly. My joints could not have loosened, and the inflammation could not have subsided so quickly. Therefore, while someone could argue that I had gone into a spontaneous remission, he would have to have an explanation for the context in which the healing was introduced and the rapidity of onset, which was more rapid than cessation of the acute inflammatory response and more rapid than improvement from any medication that I had ever taken.

In Chapter 6 we relate the story of Sally. She was ill with end stage metastatic cancer and had scan-demonstrated cancer throughout her chest, liver, bones, and abdomen. She had run the gamut of chemotherapy and radiation treatments. When Alta Ada laid hands on her in faith and prayed for her, she was within 48 hours of death. She was in septic shock and had received one treatment (of six) with a salvage chemotherapeutic agent. Salvage agents are used as a last attempt to do something for an individual, using drugs that have not been established as well as standard agents. They are usually an experimental agent. Alta Ada's friend over a 3-week period recovered from the sepsis, and her metastatic disease started to melt away. Subsequent scans showed resolution of all the previous lesions that could be identified. This healing was close to miraculous. Someone could say that perhaps the salvage agent worked. The context, the timing, and the result all speak to divine healing.

2. Background to my faith

    To understand my healing completely, one must know something about my Christian background. As a young child I attended Sunday School and church on a regular basis. It was not until during my last year of medical school that I entered into a personal relationship with God as I made a commitment to Him in exchange for the promise of eternal life. At that time I had attended church for many years on a regular basis, and I had learned a lot of facts from the Bible about God. At some level I knew that I did not have a commitment to Him, and this kept confronting me in subtle ways at various times. The issues really were not clear in my mind, because I did not dwell on them until I began to see evidence that I could not ignore. This evidence was largely through observing other people who had a long-standing relationship with God or who had recently come into relationship with God. I could sense and observe something in their lives that mine did not have. One can study a lot about a person through hearing others tell of their relationships with that person and also by reading their writings. This does not mean that one has a personal relationship with that person. It is the same in a relationship with God. Many of us know of God and about God. We must not for one minute think that this brings us into a relationship with God. When I came into a relationship with God, however, the Scriptures began to open themselves up to me in a new and very vital way.

    Soon after coming into relationship with God, I noticed that He was teaching me about Himself through His word; and He was also setting tasks for me in order for me to learn principles. Often, He would lead me to books that He wanted me to read. A Scottish physician who had been given a divine "gift of healing" had written one of these books. This doctor would get a physical discomfort in his hands sometimes when visiting a patient, and this would be a sign to him that he should lay hands on the patient and pray for his healing. He frequently would not get any such sensation, and most of the time he would practice his profession in the usual way according to those precepts that he had learned as a medical student. He wrote the book with a sense of amazement that God would work through him in this manner to bring about healing. As a new medical graduate I thought how helpful it would be for my patients if God would give me this gift also. I asked God to do so, and nothing seemed to happen; so after a while I stopped thinking about it for several years.

3.   Background to my beliefs concerning healing

I had always believed that God *could* heal people in a supernatural manner. Although I never felt that He had confined Himself to healing through natural methods such as through physicians, I really had not spent much time thinking about these issues. In fact, what little I saw of claims of healing had given me a very skeptical view of healing. In the early 1980's, for example, I had a patient with diabetes mellitus who was taking insulin. She came to me one day and told me that she would not need to come back to see me. She related to me that she had been at a service at church and had been healed by a visiting pastor. She had stopped taking her medications and insulin. I told her that it would be wise to let me check to see if she had been healed. I did not see her for some two or three years. The next time I saw her she came to see me in the emergency room with gangrene in her leg, necessitating an amputation. She had high blood glucose levels which indicated that she still had the diabetes. Gangrene is a frequent complication of out-of-control diabetes. Clearly, she had not been healed of her diabetes when she thought that she had. This left a profound concern in my mind about what she had termed "faith healing." Whatever had been implied to my patient had been untruthful and unkind, and it left her with disastrous consequences.

A friend of mine, a physician colleague, related to me on one occasion how he had been at a church service where there was a visiting healer. The healer prayed over people who had one leg shorter than the other, and before everyone's eyes people's legs were lengthened. He asked me for my thoughts, and I replied that I thought that the healer was deceiving people. Most people have mild differences in leg length, and relaxing muscles on one side while contracting them on the other could certainly appear as if a leg were being lengthened.

For these and other reasons I was neutral, if not negative, to divine healing. I had never attended any churches that taught anything about faith healing, I had seen disastrous consequences for a patient, and my colleague had related a story to me that sounded as if he had witnessed a hoax.

Alta Ada had a close friend, Susan, whose healing is recounted in Chapter 6. I did not know her when she was healed; but in speaking with her, I thought that she seemed an honest person. Her healing was attested by her nephew, who was a physician, and by other friends. I learned to value her prayers for us and her spiritual insight. I accepted that she had been healed, but I did not study the issues at that time. It did keep my mind open, however.

4. Our illnesses and the issues leading up to our healing

In my final year at medical school I was diagnosed with rheumatoid arthritis. I suffered with it for 23 years before God healed it. During those years it was reasonably stable, due to the use of medication and other treatments, until 1992 and 1993, when I had one minor flare up followed by a major flare up.

During 1993 our family was considering moving from the Boston area to Iowa. I was having a lot of pain from the arthritis and could not cope with walking the distances that I needed to walk for my work. In fact, I turned down an excellent job because I could not do the necessary walking to get to the job site. I was having severe problems with a flare up and generally felt very stiff. Many of my joints ached and remained stiff most of the day. My right ankle was particularly painful and caused me to walk in a very awkward manner. Every step I took was extremely painful. Some of the orthopedic surgeons with whom I worked had come up to me in the hall of the hospital and told me (without my solicitation) that I should have the ankle fused.

We had a friend who, in April 1992, had asked the elders of our church to lay hands on him, anoint him with oil, and pray for healing of his acute myeloid leukemia. (Evan's story is in Chapter 6.) It had gone into remission, and in late 1993 it was still in remission. This was extremely unusual to have such a prolonged remission for this type of leukemia at his age. I strongly believed that God had intervened supernaturally on his behalf. The Holy Spirit used these circumstances to have me ponder the Scriptures in James concerning healing. The Lord kept drawing me back to the Scriptures, especially James 5, and I could not get them out of my mind. As I reread the Word, my faith grew; and, while still very weak, I called my pastor and asked him if he would have the elders anoint me with oil and pray for the healing of the right ankle. In other words, this Scripture became my *rhema* for healing.

In December 1993 the elders did pray and anoint me for healing of pain in the ankle. I felt nothing during the service;

but about a week later, I realized that the pain had gone. That particular pain has never returned, although Satan seems to have tried once or twice unsuccessfully to cause it to return. I gave credit to God for healing the ankle, but even this did not lead me to study divine healing. I really did not think at that time about having prayer for the whole disease; this would have been beyond my faith at that point.

During the spring of 1995 I had come under considerable work-related stress. The arthritis was worsening, as it frequently does during periods of stress. For the first time in my life I felt my spirit was broken. The disease seemed to be taking a firm grip, and my symptoms were much worse. I felt that I was losing ground to the disease. By 1995 I was generally deteriorating in my physical abilities. I was already on six medications to treat the disease and some of the side effects of the core medications were very unpleasant. I was taking (by injection) methotrexate, a drug used in chemotherapy, which can cause cirrhosis of the liver; plaquenil, which can cause blindness; prednisone, which has well-known side effects; and other medications. The methotrexate caused me to feel nauseated and ill about half of each week. I was contemplating having to use additional medications, such as gold injections, to control the disease process with the hope of bringing it into remission, or at least stabilizing the degenerative process. My rheumatologist wanted to use increasing doses of current medications and add new ones. As a physician I was very concerned about the potential side effects of the proposed new medications. I was considering getting a motorized chair to avoid walking. My doctor did not want me to do this, as he felt that I would never walk again if I gave in at this point. I was concerned about finding work with which I could physically cope.

In addition, Alta Ada was having major physical problems from spinal stenosis that led me to take her for evaluation at the Mayo clinic. She was in constant pain, slept poorly, and could not stand for more than five minutes. I could not foresee much future for Alta Ada or me as a result of our disabilities.

I was starting for the first time in my life to think that I would not be able to reach the goals for my life for which I had been striving. I had believed, since I first came to know God personally, that He was preparing me for a ministry. I had not seen a definite focus for this ministry, but it was a deeply held conviction in my spirit that it would involve teaching about being led by the Holy Spirit. I was beginning to feel that I would not be able to manage physically to do those things that I was sure were a part of God's plan for me. I was in moderate despair about the two of us with our physical infirmities during the first half of 1995. I would sit for periods of time praying about the situation, but not once did I ask God to heal us. That may seem strange in view of the healing that I am about to relate. My focus, however, was more on grieving a loss of health and just expressing this grief to God. I also was asking Him at that time to bring us into a work that we could share together. During the early part of 1995 a friend in Florida whom we had never met but with whom we had developed a friendship and spiritual communion *via* telephone and mail invited us to come to visit him. We prayed about the timing of such a trip, and the time did not seem to be right.

During the middle of the summer I was driving in my car alone. I had been musing about some work I had been doing in a library in a nearby town. I was on my way home and praying about some of the things that I had been reading. Suddenly God spoke to me, stating, "You have much to learn yet." This was not the first time that God had spoken to me like this. When it happens, one is filled instinctively with the knowledge of what God is addressing. I knew that this related to our pending trip to visit our friends in Florida. This word was a *rhema*, spoken directly by God. Our friend once more asked us to come, this time on a particular date. We acted on it; and as we planned for the trip, both of our spirits were filled with an increasing expectation that God was going to do something in our lives. We still were not thinking of healing. Even as we drove down to Florida, our aches and pains accompanied us.

5. The healing announced

While in Florida in September 1995 we attended four church services over a three-day period. Three of these services had prophetic ministry. This was new to us, and in each of these three services the prophetic teams ministered to us. While we were there, a prophetic presbytery (as mentioned in 1 Timothy 4:14) prayed over me and told me that I would be healed as I walked. (We have a record of one of Jesus' healings in this way— the ten men with leprosy reported in Luke 17:11-19.) The Lord indicated through the ministry teams that He was healing me of rheumatoid arthritis and that He was healing Alta Ada of spinal stenosis. It was a total surprise. When Alta Ada awakened the next morning, she had lost the feeling of a heavy weight dragging her down as she stood. (Alta Ada relates this story in Chapter 3.) At one of the services the elders of one of the churches anointed me with oil and prayed for healing. Within days I was able to break into almost a run. This was something that I had not been able to do for years.

RA (rheumatoid arthritis) is a disease of the immune system, and its activity can be measured by blood tests. For twenty years my blood tests for the RA factor had been at least 1:1280. This means that when one part of my blood was diluted with 1280 parts of something else, the RA factor was still strong enough to be detected. Technically, there should be none in the blood; but, since many things can put traces in the blood, a reading of 1:40 is considered normal. Two weeks and one day after these two services, I had my blood tested. *My blood titer measured 1:80!* God had indeed healed me.

Within a week of the services our next door neighbor, a physical therapist, observed me almost running. This was something I had not been able to do for several years. During the fall of that year I was able to remove the leaves from our entire yard. This would have been impossible previously. I had not taken any of the methotrexate since one week after leaving Florida, and I planned to taper off the other three primary medications gradually.

After the immediate event and after we expressed our thankfulness to God for what He had given us, we started to meditate about the situation. Clearly God had shown us with evidence that was internally and externally convincing that He was still in the business of healing people of physical ailments in this life.

The physical improvement from the healing was observed by a number of friends, professionals, and family. I was excited about what God had given to us, and I wanted to let people know about it. However, I had a great restraint about talking about God's healing me due to the fact that I knew of people who had wanted healing and had not received it. It seemed unkind to talk about it before developing a deeper understanding of why God had chosen to heal me. Also I wanted to consider carefully how to integrate this new revelation into my professional life. God is not one to play favorites, and also He is not one to make us earn something such as healing. It is a gift, just like salvation, since the Lord Jesus Christ paid for it by the events surrounding the crucifixion. We, therefore, cannot earn it; nor can we deserve it. We can ask for it just as we can ask for salvation.

One of the things that God used to convince me of the truth of the prophetic ministry was that the prophets spoke things to me that I had not shared even with Alta Ada. These were things concerning future ministry dreams. These prophets were absolutely correct. The morning and afternoon after the first service I was emotionally stunned. Essentially, God had opened up a whole new revelation of Himself to us. It meant revisiting concepts that we had taken as truth. It meant relearning a lot of Scripture. God had been absolutely correct with what He had said to me as I had been driving in the car a few weeks earlier: I did still have much to learn.

As a physician I was amazed to note the changes in my body. I was too awed yet even to be thinking about the whole situation; but my joints were loosened, pain was lessened, and I was feeling better. This in no way was a psychological hyping up or an emotional fake. My mind was examining everything with a critical edge, while my emotions were stunned.

God had spoken a very compelling *rhema* into both of our lives concerning healing. He had accentuated it by repeating it three times with different prophetic teams in a very short space of time. Obviously it was very important to Him and to us that we should believe it.

6.   The devil's counterattack

After I received healing for about six or eight weeks, I was able to move my joints very freely. I felt very well. Then the symptoms of joint pain and stiffness began to return. I did not understand what was happening, but the events motivated me both to study God's Word and to read every book that I could find that had been written about faith healing. Most of the books concentrated on the actual healing in isolation of the circumstances leading to it and the follow up from it. There was little that I could find about maintaining a healing that God had given. One author who dealt with this issue was Kenneth E. Hagin. He had experienced God's healing himself; and he was able to write with insight, having been healed and also having ministered in healing.

Through reading books, studying the Bible, praying, and pondering, I began to see that God had healed me and that what was now occurring was a counterattack from the devil. The devil and his agents were trying to undo the work that God had done in my body. After being healed, I had been praying about what I should do about my medications. I had continued on most of them, and now as I was experiencing rapid worsening of my physical situation I kept taking them. As a trained medical professional I was able to note that the new symptoms I was experiencing were very similar to the old ones but subtly different. I am unsure that a non-professional would have been able to make the distinction. [I have since come to believe that Satan either cannot or does not put the original disease back upon someone who is healed, but he can and does put symptoms that are similar. Only when we open a door through rebellion toward God or through unbelief and doubt does the original disease return. See the fuller discussion in Chapter 4.]

I had received the healing in early September 1995 and felt very well six to eight weeks. In early 1996 I was desperately trying to decide what I should do about the sudden deterioration in my health. I found myself probably worse than before the healing. In reading God's Word, I noted that the Lord Jesus had never said, "No," to anyone who came to Him directly and asked for healing. He is the same yesterday, today, and forever; so that meant to me that He was willing to heal me. I began to study the Scriptures that had been so important to Kenneth E. Hagin when he had been healed. This was Mark 11:23–24. I studied Scriptures on faith. I understood that Jesus had already paid for my healing and that I had to appropriate it by faith.

In grappling with understanding God and how He deals with healing, I found that no one author was really explaining the process of faith healing in a way that I could understand it. Many authors had an emphasis on faith, but no one seemed to be explaining how one acquired faith for healing. Some authors seemed to be implying that if we believed in healing, then we would have it. I believed in healing, but mine was slipping away. I did not know how I could believe "more" than I did. The idea of mustering up faith by believing God's word troubled me. It was almost as if some people were saying that if a person believes God's word tenaciously enough, then by "naming it and claiming it" he commits God to fulfilling His Word. This bothered me, since it could leave God out of the healing loop or, for that matter, any other area of faith that an individual approached in that manner. Clearly, God tells us that He is the healer. Therefore, God has to be involved individually in healing a person when faith healing is involved. At that time I did not get all of the facts sorted out, but God dealt graciously with me by leading me to study the Scriptures about Abraham.

In studying Abraham's life I was struck by how difficult it would be for me to believe God for a child at the ages Abraham and Sarah were. I did not know it at that time, but in retrospect this was God's *rhema* to me to start me walking in faith based on His previous *rhemas* to me about giving me healing. He was showing me that He had promised healing to me in His Word (*logos*). He had told me *via* several prophets independently over a short period that He had healed me (*rhema*). Just as God had expected Abraham to walk in belief about the child, He was now testing me to see if I would walk in belief that I was healed. This was Mark 11:23-24 coming into action. It came only after I received both the *logos* and then the *rhema*. "Faith comes by hearing and hearing by the Word (*rhema*) of God" (Romans 10:17). Chapter 10 elaborates on this process.

I decided to stop my medications, despite getting worse physically. As a physician I knew how to do this in a way that would not be life-threatening. While I might get worse, I would not lose my life. I gradually stopped my medications; and, surely enough, I got worse. For several months I could not pull even a sheet up over myself. I was very weak. I would come down stairs once a day very slowly and go back up slowly later in the evening. I was not able to stay up very long. I kept on singing the refrain to myself, "I come, Lord, without one plea except, Dear Lord, that you died for me." I had an absolute bedrock belief that I had been healed. This was due to God's *logos*, followed by His *rhema*, having been placed into my spirit. I knew that I had been healed, and from Kenneth E. Hagin's writings I knew that the devil and his agents were trying to undo the healing. I knew that God was expecting me to stand on His Word, just as He expected Abraham to stand on it.

Gradually I began to stabilize, and my joints improved. I gradually recovered strength. I was able to resume practicing medicine in a less physically demanding setting in the fall of 1996. Gradually I was able to increase my activities, until in early 2000 I was able to get back to a regular practice schedule that has meant 12-hour days.

Several times the devil and his agents have tried to frighten me with return of similar symptoms; but it is increasingly easy to call this for what it is, pay it no attention, and continue with discomfort for a few days. It soon disappears. I did have one major flare-up a few years ago. That was for a particular purpose that God was working in our lives. God has used these attacks from the enemy to teach me some principles about spiritual warfare and faith. What the devil intends for harm God will always use for good. When one has a victory in the Lord, Satan always attacks.

7. Post-healing challenges

Following God's healing us in these areas of physical disability, we were faced with several challenges. Many of the people we knew were not familiar with healing and were pleased for us that we had been healed. However, we knew that God's Word clearly explains that He does not play favorites; therefore, since He healed us, there must be access to any other believer for healing. We wanted to understand faith healing in order to explain it to others and to help them.

I was faced with what to tell patients about faith healing. I had the negative impressions from earlier; but now that God had given me healing, I had to come to an understanding of how God interacts with His created people in this area. Lacking a full under-standing, I settled for telling people that it was no different to the times that Jesus walked about on the earth with His ministry. I felt myself to be on solid ground with this explanation. I did not want to be in the position of having anyone deceived as my earlier patient had been. Of course I was not involved in a healing ministry, but rather the practice of medicine. It has been very encouraging to many people, both acquaintances and patients, to let them know that God still heals.

By telling people that obtaining faith healing is no different now to how it was during Jesus' ministry, I was on solid ground because of the *logos*. I had no problem with the following explanation since it left the hearer in a position of having to approach the Lord Jesus for healing. I would explain that God tells us that He is the same yesterday, today, and forever. Therefore His nature will not change. It was Jesus' will to heal all who came to Him in faith, believing that He was willing and able to heal. Therefore, if one will go to the Lord in prayer and ask to be healed, then that healing will be given in due time if the person has gone in faith. He must approach Jesus both believing that He is able to heal him and that He is willing to heal him. He must wait on and plead with Him, just as the Syrophoenecian woman had to plead and wait. He must tarry until he gets his *rhema*. It may be that he will have to wrestle with the Lord just as Jacob did. It is only when he obtains the *rhema* that he knows that he has been given healing. Notice that it was only after I received my *rhema* from the story of Abraham and Sarah that I was able to stand against the devil and keep the healing that the Lord had given to me.

Based on the Scripture I believe that a person unwilling to commit his life to the Lord may well be able to prevail upon Him for healing, but I do not see a legal basis for being able to expect it. We should expect the healing process to be the same as the salvation process. There has to be a personal meaningful interaction with the Lord for both salvation and healing. One caveat is that for both we must come empty handed in our spirit with no pretension of earning or deserving either healing or salvation.

8. Further healing

Since receiving the initial healing both Alta Ada and I have been placed in several situations by the Lord that have required healing for us or for a friend or family member. We tell some of these stories throughout this book. One word that the Lord spoke to us in Florida in 1995 was that no disease or infirmity could cling to us. We believed that word and have based several decisions on it. It was a *rhema* to us.

We began to see that God would like to use us in ministry to some degree in the area of healing. Perhaps that is part of why we started to get various health problems. I have had problems at times with chest pains, a probable cancer on an eyelid, and an irregular heartbeat. In addition, the changes from the rheumatoid arthritis when it was active have left me with degenerative joint problems in my knees. All of these issues I have left in trust for the Lord to deal with in His own time. I have not sought Him for immediate healing except for the cancer. In this case I asked Him if He wanted me to have surgery, or if He would take care of it. I had an immediate vision of the lesion drying up and dropping off. My pastor had the same vision without knowing the answer that I had received. Out of the mouths of two or three witnesses these things are established. I did not spend any time worrying any further about this situation; and a few years later, when I had to see a doctor about another small growth on my face, he confirmed that the lesion was gone.

Alta Ada has been challenged by several bouts of irregular heartbeats (atrial fibrillation) that are quite fatiguing and uncomfortable. With these there is an immediate need for resolution, and so we pray for these to be healed each time they occur. The Lord has normalized the irregularity on each occasion. As a physician it is very stressful for me to know of all potential complications of irregular heartbeats, as I have to wait in faith on God to resolve it. One very interesting *rhema* that I received on it occurred on an occasion when the problem had been going on for more than 24 hours. We had prayed, but no healing had occurred. I was busy moving some of our belongings from an apartment to our newly-purchased home. A physician friend of ours telephoned and talked with Alta Ada. He was concerned for her and telephoned me to urge me to take her to the emergency room. I have always offered to do that for her, but she has not felt that she should do that.

I decided that this time I should take her, since the problem had gone on for so long. While driving the ten minutes to the house I was praying about it. The Lord spoke a *rhema* to me. He said to me quite clearly "If I should choose not to heal Alta Ada, why would you wish to get her healed?" I was absolutely shocked by this. I knew that God had not said that He wouldn't heal her, but He was challenging me with something of far greater depth.

When I got to Alta Ada, I said to her that I would take her to the hospital. I was not being disobedient, but I had to think through what God had just said to me. Now when I told her that I would take her to the hospital she said, "Feel my pulse and if it is not regular, I'll go." She had just received a word of wisdom (*rhema*) from God that it would be regular. After more than 24 hours the heart reverted to normal right at that time. Even when she made the statement, she had not had a regular heartbeat. As I have pondered my lack of faith in this issue, I look at God's amazing timing. I had waited for a long time without trying to get Alta Ada to the hospital, but I finally had given in to peer pressure. God is a very gentle teacher, and He used this episode to show how closely He is working with us and how detail-oriented He is even to the precise second on the timing. Alta Ada has since had many *rhemas* telling her that God will give her a complete healing in this area.

9.   A broken hip

In September 2003 we had returned to Florida for a church conference at the location where we had first received prophecy about healing. I do not know the reasons why; but on the trip to Florida, as I was driving, I was musing before the Lord about the various things from which He had healed me. I had been healed from respiratory viruses, tooth pain, and the rheumatoid arthritis. I had no complications of a bad bout of chest pain. My heart had regularized from an abnormal rhythm. I began to think about what the Lord would do for me, if I had an acute injury such as a broken bone.

Two days later after leaving the first evening session of the conference, I fell on uneven ground at the edge of the parking lot. I just lost my balance and fell onto grass. I found that I could not get up. I had suffered a fracture through the neck of the femur. I was transported by ambulance to a local hospital and admitted for treatment.

I prayed and asked the Lord if He was going to heal me or whether I should have surgery. I discussed the situation with the pastors of the local church the next morning. The senior pastor gave me very wise counsel. He essentially advised me to be ruled by peace. If I felt at peace about the surgery, then that should be fine. In a situation like that, it is hard to look into the spirit and discern whether there is peace, because there are all sorts of emotions in the soul. Nonetheless, I felt that there was an internal peace about having surgery. Later that evening I underwent surgery (a total hip replacement) for the fracture.

As I look back on the incident, I see that it would have been very difficult for me to wait on the Lord. I did not really wait for a *rhema*. I do not know if the Lord would have given me a miraculous healing. I may never know the answer to that question. Some of the factors that pressured me into making a decision for surgery were the risk of complications that would increase the longer I waited, the difficulty of explaining to my insurance company that I was waiting on the Lord before deciding about surgery, the emotional numbness related to the injury, and the fatigue that I was experiencing. In addition, we were more than 1000 miles from our home; we had no way to stay in the area longer; and we had no way to be transported back to our home area for surgery that was feasible.

After surgery I had confidence to ask the Lord to heal me rapidly without complications. After six weeks I was able to go back to work on a half time basis. I was working full time within twelve weeks with no complications. During the week in the hospital I found that being a physician really is not fun, as one knows the potential complications of a condition. The devil attacked my mind and emotions relentlessly. He and his agents tried to convince me that I would die of a complication. I refuted the arguments and refused to listen. It was still a very wearying time; the devil will frequently attack when one is weak. The Lord protected me, and I realized anew just how much we have to rely on the Lord to preserve us in this life, when we are exposed to the hatred of the enemy.

10. Fighting against the enemy

I have noticed when I am seeing someone with a bad contagious disease such as a respiratory virus that the devil's agents will try to put a picture in my mind of my becoming ill with it. The insertion is so subtle that one might not even notice it if one were not paying attention to it. If I agree to that picture and entertain it, then almost surely the infection will be transmitted.

Once I understood this and talked with Alta Ada about this, she realized that this had happened to her on many occasions. One type of occasion is when she would get a "scratchy" throat or a little nasal drainage. Previously, she had pictured herself under the bed covers, suffering with the cold, and waiting for it to pass. This "picture" always was a self-fulfilling prophecy. She began to reject that picture upon getting a symptom and to seek the Lord and ask for healing, and usually the illness has not materialized. It can be a wearying battle, however.

One has to practice waging a war against the enemy in the mind and emotions. We are instructed to take every thought captive for the Lord. This means learning to examine every thought for the source. If we reject those from the enemy and those from our own imaginations that build ourselves up, then we will indeed be able to renew our minds; and we will be able to stand and resist the enemy in a variety of decisions and circumstances that may well be a prelude to illness.

The practice of this takes time. It will be a process that requires patience and perseverance. These are qualities that the Lord wants to see in our spirits. The Lord will surely help us, as we ask Him to train us in this transformation of our minds.

11. Patience

On some occasions the Lord seems to heal instantly when we ask. This has happened for us as we have laid hands on a sore eye for Alta Ada. Other times He makes us wait for months after we ask for healing. We have to step back and see that we have a very impatient, self-centered approach to healing. If it hurts, we want it stopped. The Lord sees the whole picture for our lives, and He is trying to bring us to maturity in our souls so that we can rule and reign with Him in the ages to come.

He also is weaving everything together for good in the life of every believer. Everything means *everything* (every molecule and every second is accounted for in the lives of millions of people for eternity). This requires genius on a scale that our minds cannot begin to fathom. God tells us: "For *as* the heavens are higher than the earth, so are my ways higher than your ways, and my thoughts than your thoughts" (Isaiah 55:9). The man beside the Pool of Siloam (John 9) had done no wrong. His parents had done no wrong. He had to wait for his healing until it was the time for God to be glorified (v.3). God is glorified when we patiently suffer **for His purposes** (not for our doings) and He is also glorified when we hang tenaciously to His promise of healing. If He allows the promise of healing to tarry, it will be for a complexity of reasons that we do not understand. That does not mean that we will not be healed. Abraham had to wait years before his *rhema* was fulfilled. Part of it was not fulfilled in his lifetime. We have to be patient. It is an essential fruit of the spirit that we have to acquire to mature.

God is not in the business of providing instant gratification to us. That would leave us as spiritual babes. Faith is proven as we wait. When we see someone else healed, we have no idea of how long he may have had to wait. In addition, God expects us to pursue our requests to Him with vigor. He is not interested in our being double minded (James 1:6-8). If we want healing, we have to request it and keep after it. It may be that God will wish to make changes in our lives before healing us. This may make it easier for us to accept a healing in the right way. When we ask God for healing, we have to believe that we have it when we ask (Mark 11:23-24). We get this belief by getting a *rhema* from God. However, the actual physical manifestations may require a series of changes in our attitudes and beliefs in order for the healing to occur. Once we ask the Lord to heal us when we have faith to receive it, then if the healing tarries, we must ask the Lord what we should do in order to prepare for it.

When I was healed of the rheumatoid arthritis, the Lord also told me that I would have no infirmity that could cling to me. I believe that, but I still have all of the deformities in my hands and other joints that 22 years of rheumatoid activity left. I believe that the Lord will eventually restore these joints to functionality according to the *rhema*. In the meantime the deformities have led a number of patients, friends, and other people to ask me questions concerning what happened to my hands or if I hurt. Those questions give me a very easy introduction to telling the story of how the Lord heals. I am quite content to wait on the *rhema* to be fulfilled. I have no doubt that it will be fulfilled. In the meantime God is using the situation to speak to others He places in contact with me. This is one example of how the Lord is working many things at any instant to bring good to all of His people all of the time.

12. Hope versus faith

This is a critical area to understand if one is going to receive divine healing. Hebrews 11:1 states that "faith is the substance of things hoped for, the evidence of things not seen." Chapter 4 examines this verse in greater detail. Thus, one can hope for something; but when he gets a *rhema* that he knows is from God, he can trust it; and this is faith. This book deals with this concept in more detail in Chapter 10 in the section on obtaining the *rhema*.

One evening while driving home from work I was talking to the Lord and asking Him why more people do not receive healing from Him. He indicated to me that people with illness will come to Him for healing but do not usually know Him well enough to develop the required faith.

The essence of developing faith is obtaining the ability to know the Lord's voice so that we can distinguish when He speaks to us, when we hear from our own soul, and when Satan and his demons speak to us. Distinguishing these different voices and manners of speaking takes some practice and time. We must develop a close relationship with God to accomplish this. When Jesus walked the earth, people would go to Him and thus know that He was talking with them. We need just the same knowledge today.

When we know God's voice from experience and when we hear Him tell us that He will heal us, then we are in a very strong position to withstand the faith-weakening efforts of the devil to plant doubt. We can certainly expect him to do this.

Section IV

8
Answers to Objections to Healing

There are several arguments that some people advance to try to prove that God is not healing in the church today. They fall into two categories.

There are those who say that all miracles have ceased, that God does not heal today. Some of these people will say that they believe that God *can* heal (they almost have to confess this if they do not deny the omnipotence of God), but they think He chooses not to do so.

There are more people who, by and large, do not think of God healing today but believe that God sometimes heals. They look on this healing as sporadic, almost on a whim. They look at healing as something upon which we cannot count, and they think we cannot know whether to expect healing in a given situation. They would tend to end prayers for healing with "if it be in Thy will." They really do not understand God's healing character.

Those Who Believe All Miracles Have Ceased

We will deal with the former group first. Many of the people in this group claim that miracle gifts ceased sometime in the first century, depending on which of several dates they accept. They group healing in this category. (There are cessationists [as these people are called, since they believe that miracles have ceased] who think that healing still occurs, although they would say that prophecy, tongues, and other miracles have ceased.)

The cessationists give several dates for the ending of these miracles. Some say that these gifts were used only by the apostles;

and with the death of John (the last apostle to die) around 100 A.D., they ceased. We can point to many Scriptures, however, showing that non-apostles had these gifts: the deacon Stephen—great wonders and miracles, Acts 6:8; the deacon and evangelist Philip—miracles and healing of palsy, lameness, and demon possession, Acts 8:6-7; Ananias—no particular office, healing of the blindness of Saul of Tarsus, Acts 9:17-18; Agabus—prophecy, Acts 11:28 and Acts 21:10-11; Judas and Silas—prophecy, Acts 15:32; and four daughters of Philip—prophecy, Acts 21:9.

Not only do the Scriptures name many who were not apostles who had these gifts, but the Bible also specifically states that all believers should be able to function in some of these areas: "And these signs shall follow **them that believe**; In my name shall they cast out devils; they shall speak with new tongues; They shall take up serpents; and if they drink any deadly thing, it shall not hurt them; they shall lay hands on the sick, and they shall recover" (Mark 16:17-18—emphasis ours). Thus, this argument fails.

There are other theories, however. Some give the date of the destruction of the temple, 70 A.D., for the cessation of sign gifts. There is no Biblical basis for this. Some state that "that which is perfect" (see next paragraph) is the canon of Scripture, and they argue for cessation of these gifts about 95 A.D. with the writing of The Revelation. Again, there is no linguistic or other basis that this phrase "that which is perfect" refers to the completion of the canon of Scripture. Most likely, this refers either to the Eternal State, when the perfect atmosphere and society will be set up, or to the time when Jesus returns to set up His perfect kingdom. At any rate, neither interpretation would support the argument for these gifts' not being operative today; and, in addition, as noted below, this passage does not refer to healing.

Many of the people who say that healing is not intended for today's church will quote 1 Corinthians 13:8-10: "Love never faileth: but whether *there be* prophecies, they shall fail; whether *there be* tongues, they shall cease; whether *there be* knowledge, it shall vanish away. For we know in part, and we prophesy in part. But when that which is perfect is come, then that which is in part shall be done away." They say that tongues, prophecy, healing, and other miracle gifts have ceased. An interesting thing about using this passage is that it names prophecies, tongues, and word of knowledge—three of the spiritual gifts. It does not address healing; therefore, regardless of the interpretation of the passage, one cannot interpret it to indicate cessation of healing.

Thus, all the arguments for the cessation of healings sometime in the first century fail. These all rely on some criterion for setting some date for cessation. All of them overlook a very important part of any discussion on healing—the character of God, which we discussed in Chapter 1. It is not consistent with the compassionate, healing, caring God to heal people from ancient Old Testament times through the first century of this era, only to stop and leave His people without hope for healing in this age.

Many cessationists try to show in some way that even the apostle Paul could no longer heal toward the end of his life. A reading of Acts 28:8-9 shows that Paul, after healing the father of Publius, healed apparently all on the island of Melita (Malta) who came to him for healing. Certainly at this time, late in his life, Paul shows no signs of having lost the power to heal.

These cessationists will sometimes point to various Scriptures showing that someone is sick (*e.g.*, Trophimus—2 Timothy 4:20). There are several answers other than that Paul no longer had the power to heal. Since not everyone avails himself of healing today, we might expect that not everyone exercised his faith in Paul's day.

Probably the most quoted passage in this respect is 1 Timothy 5:23 in which Paul advises Timothy to drink water no longer, but to drink wine for the frequent infirmities of his stomach. This type of advice we will cover in Chapter 10. Here we will just state the principle that it is always wise to take care of our bodies in any way we can. Thus, if we know of an inherent weakness in our bodies, we should eat, exercise, or rest in ways that do not stress this area. To plunge recklessly ahead in any lifestyle, expecting God to rescue us from disaster, is to "jump from the pinnacle of the temple," metaphorically. Jesus' response to Satan, when he so tempted Him, was that we should not tempt the Lord, Our God.

Thus, we have seen that none of the arguments of the cessationists stand up under the scrutiny of Scriptures. Most of the people who argue that signs, including healing, have ceased have a belief that they can articulate very clearly. They hold to a very dry orthodoxy in which God does not interact in the lives of His people.

Those Who Do Not Understand God's Healing Character

The second group of people who do not avail themselves of God's healing contains most of the typical churchgoers (as opposed to theologians) who do not understand God's healing today. They primarily do not believe in healing because they have not been taught. They tend to be very timid about approaching God with promises; thus, they do not claim the healing promises in prayer. We will discuss the problems with or objections to healing that occur in this second group of people.

When To Pray "Thy Will Be Done"

Many people tend to end their prayers with that great faith-killer, "Thy will be done." Now, it is very important to understand the use of this phrase. Certainly, there is a legitimate use for praying, "Thy will be done." Our Lord set the example for this in His agony in the garden of Gethsemane. We are to pray this phrase in the following cases:

1. when we do not know God's will in a particular situation,
2. when we would like God to change His mind or when we do not like what God is asking us to do but are willing to submit to His plan, or
3. when we are directly calling down God's foreordained program.

When we do not know God's will in a particular situation, we can pray to know God's will and to do God's will. David tells us that we can ask God to show us which way to go: "What man is he that feareth the Lord? Him shall he teach in the way that he shall choose" (Psalm 25:12) and "I will instruct thee and teach thee in the way which thou shalt go; I will guide thee with mine eye" (Psalm 32:8). James states that "if any of you lack wisdom, let him ask of God, who giveth to all men liberally, and upbraideth not, and it shall be given him" (James 1:5). When we pray this way, we are, in effect, praying for God's will. An example of this type of situation would be in looking for a job. We might not have had a direct word from God about what job to take; we would pray, asking God to show us and saying, "Let Your will be done in the situation." In other words, we use that phrase to let God know we are willing to do whatever He wants of us.

The perfect example of the second category above is that of our Lord. In Gethsemane Jesus was expressing His own agony.

He was saying that He did not want to go to the cross, in His own heart. But, knowing that it was God's will for Him to go to the cross to accomplish our salvation, He submitted to God, saying, "Not my will but thine be done."

One example of the third category is found in the model prayer. When Jesus instructs us to pray "...thy will be done on earth as it is in heaven," we are praying for God's kingdom to come to earth. This is in God's foreordained plan, but we do not know the timing. Thus, when we pray this prayer, we are asking for God's plan to be set in motion.

This is much the same type of prayer that Daniel prayed. Daniel, from a study of the Scriptures, realized that the seventy-year period of captivity was nearly over. He began to pray for God to effect His plan for Israel, *i.e.*, for God's will to be done. He tells us, "...I, Daniel, understood by books the number of the years, concerning which the word of the Lord came to Jeremiah, the prophet, that he would accomplish seventy years in the desolations of Jerusalem. And I set my face unto the Lord God, to seek by prayer and supplications, with fasting, and sackcloth, and ashes....O Lord...defer not, for thine own sake, O my God; for thy city and thy people are called by thy name" (Daniel 9:2-3,19). Thus, he was praying for God's will, that is, God's revealed plan for Israel, to be accomplished.

One very effective way to pray in any situation, not just for healing, is to go into God's presence and to ask Him how He wants us to pray in that situation. After we hear from God, we then know His will in that area. With confidence we can pray very particularly and pray for God's will to be done, as we know what His will is. We have done that on several occasions and have found the prayer in this manner to be very powerful and effective.

When we are not to pray, "Thy will be done" is when we already know God's will. For example, we have never heard anyone pray for someone's salvation in this way, "Dear Lord, I pray that Jane will be saved. Nevertheless, let this happen only if it is in your will." We know that "God is not willing that any should perish" (2 Peter 3:9); thus, we do not pray that way. Similarly, we know that it is not God's will for any believer to marry an unbeliever (2 Corinthians 6:14 and other Scriptures by inference). We should never pray, "Dear Lord, please let me marry Jane, who is an unbeliever, if it be Your will." We already know that it is not God's will. Since we have learned that it *is* God's will that we be healed, we should not pray for healing with the indefinite "if it be Your will." We have already seen that the author of Hebrews tells us that "But without faith *it is* impossible to please *him*" (11:6). Thus, it is not pleasing to God for a believer to pray for healing in that way.

In addition to not understanding the proper use of the phrase "If it be Your will," many people use other ideas to resist healing. Several of these will be considered.

Paul's Thorn in the Flesh

Some people cite the case of Paul's so-called "thorn in the flesh." The Scripture that is involved in this argument is 2 Corinthians 12:1-10. After telling of being caught up into the third heaven, the place of the throne room of God, Paul says that God inflicted him in this manner to keep him from boasting:

> [6]For though I would desire to glory, I shall not be a fool; for I will say the truth: but *now* I forbear, lest any man should think of me above that which he seeth me *to be*, or *that* he heareth of me. [7]And lest I should be exalted above measure through the abundance of the revelations, there was given to me a thorn in the flesh, the messenger

of Satan to buffet me, lest I should be exalted above measure. ⁸For this thing I besought the Lord thrice, that it might depart from me. ⁹And he said unto me, My grace is sufficient for thee: for my strength is made perfect in weakness. Most gladly therefore will I rather glory in my infirmities, that the power of Christ may rest upon me. ¹⁰Therefore I take pleasure in infirmities, in reproaches, in necessities, in persecutions, in distresses for Christ's sake: for when I am weak, then am I strong.

The word translated "messenger" is really the Greek word ἄγγελος, or *angelos*, which means "angel." It is used 186 times in the New Testament, and it is translated "angel" 179 times. Since angels were frequently messengers for God, it occasionally (seven times in the NT) was translated messenger. The word translated "infirmities" connotes the idea of weakness, not illness especially. People who have used this passage to say that Paul could not heal himself (and then they reason that healing must have stopped) fail to understand these words. Apparently, God sent, or allowed, a demon to afflict Paul's body in some irritating fashion (as a thorn would be an irritant, but not fatal) at one point in his life in order to keep him from boasting about the visions he had seen. Those people who use this text to prove cessation of healing normally overlook one key Scripture. Whatever the demon inflicted upon Paul, it seems to have been gone by the close of his life. Paul tells us that "Persecution, affliction...what persecutions I endured, but out of them **all** the Lord delivered me" (2 Timothy 3:11—emphasis ours).

Suffering for the Lord

Then there are those people who say that we must suffer for the Lord. Certainly, this is true. Passages such as John 15:18-21; John 16:33; 1 Peter 1:6-7; and 1 Peter 4:12-16 indicate that we must suffer as believers. None of these passages, however, indicate that these sufferings involve illness. In fact, when Paul listed the sufferings he had endured for Christ, illness was not one of them:

> Are they ministers of Christ? (I speak as a fool) I *am* more; in labours more abundant, in stripes above measure, in prisons more frequent, in deaths oft. Of the Jews five times received I forty *stripes* save one. Thrice was I beaten with rods, once was I stoned, thrice I suffered shipwreck, a night and a day I have been in the deep; *In* journeyings often, *in* perils of waters, *in* perils of robbers, *in* perils by *mine own* countrymen, *in* perils by the heathen, *in* perils in the city, *in* perils in the wilderness, *in* perils in the sea, *in* perils among false brethren; In weariness and painfulness, in watchings often, in hunger and thirst, in fastings often, in cold and nakedness.   2 Corinthians 11:23-27

Thus, we can expect suffering for the cause of Christ, but it will not come in the form of illness. The author of Hebrews tells us, "Though he were a Son, yet learned he obedience by the things which he suffered" (Hebrews 5:8). If God the Son had to learn obedience through suffering, none of us sinful men dare expect less. There is no indication, however, that Jesus was ever ill. God had to "make him sick" (Isaiah 53:10 [see discussion in Chapter 2]) on the cross as He atoned for sin and illness.

Sin and Illness

We should note that the Bible is consistent with showing that sometimes the result of sin is illness. This is discussed more fully in Chapter 9. Here we will just mention that many, many times the Israelites were told in the Old Testament times that certain illnesses had come upon them because of their sins (see examples in next chapter). Paul indicates that many of the Corinthians were sick and some had died due to sin at the communion table (1 Corinthians 11:30). Furthermore, God relates physical health with walking in His commandments in the very passage in which He reveals Himself as the Great Healer: "...If thou wilt diligently hearken to the voice of the Lord thy God, and wilt do that which is right in his sight, and wilt give ear to his commandments, and keep all his statutes, I will put none of these diseases upon thee, which I have brought upon the Egyptians; for I am the Lord that healeth thee" (Exodus 15:26). We will see the necessity of confession of all known sin before seeking healing in Chapter 10.

Illness as Glorification of God

Occasionally, we hear someone say something like, "God is being glorified by my illness." This idea is never presented in the Bible. In fact, Jesus tells us, "The thief cometh not but to steal, and to kill, and to destroy; I am come that they might have life, and that they might have it more abundantly" (John 10:10). God is glorified by life. Satan is the author of sin, death, and illness. He loves to inflict these on God's children. We must not let him steal, kill, and destroy what things are ours as children of God—life and health.

The Case of Job

A related objection involves the case of Job. Some people say that God was glorified by Job's suffering. An in-depth study of Job will show that God was not glorified by Job's illness; He was glorified by Job's faith. Job did not compromise when all his counselors/ friends were telling him other things. He did not deny God when his own wife advised him to curse God and die. Ezekiel groups Job with Daniel and Noah as men whom God calls righteous—implying justified by their faith (Ezekiel 14:14, 20). Thus, it is for faith that Job is acclaimed by God.

The Place of Physicians in Healing

One frequently hears someone say something like, "I believe that God heals through physicians." This brings up the question as to what place physicians have in healing. This statement is usually made by individuals who have never considered the claims of God for healing. It is a way of *seemingly* attributing healing to God without having to face the questions with which we have been dealing in this book.

In reality, the believer operating in total faith probably does not need a physician. We personally know of people who carry no health insurance and who have never needed physicians for themselves or their children. In the United States and much of the Western world believers have been so weak in this area that few are able to avail themselves completely of this provision of God. We tend to mix faith and medicine. We know people who have talked with believers in Burma and India who have raised people from the dead. It *may* be that where there is less medical help in some remote places, the believers find themselves thrust totally on the mercy of God.

The writers of the Bible accepted physicians. We see Paul referring to Luke as the "beloved physician" (Colossians 4:14). There is no condemnation of his profession. The physician certainly *should* be a person filled with the compassion of the Lord. Since most people either are not believers or are not able to believe God for healing, there is a place in our society for compassionate health care workers to try to alleviate suffering as much as they can. This is an example of God's common grace in society.

There should be no stigma on a Christian who chooses to use medical help. Since God has provided for medical help as part of His common grace, it is to be received with thanksgiving if one desires to use it. We are just suggesting that ideally God intends us to avail ourselves of what He has provided by special grace, His divine healing.

In Chapter 6 we related the Sally's story. She had metastatic cancer that had spread to most of her organs, including the liver. Her physician expected her to live less than a month, when she contracted pneumonia; this shortened her expected lifespan to two weeks. I began laying hands on her, anointing her with oil, and praying for healing at least twice a day. She was too sick to do much except agree. She believed that God wanted to heal her. Miraculously, He did! At that point, the doctors had discontinued chemotherapy, saying that it would do no good. She was not strong enough in her faith in this miracle to stop treatment at once, and she decided to have one more treatment. As we prayed about it, the Lord let us know that He had healed her and that it was irrelevant whether she had another treatment. It would not hurt her, nor would it help. Actually, when a scan showed that no cancer remained in her body, her HMO did a second scan, because they could not believe the results. The doctors told her that it looked as if there were scars from having the cancer surgically removed (she had not had surgery for this). Thus, God did not condemn her use of medicine; but He was the healer.

We should keep in mind, however, that the best physician is only treating symptoms. As we quoted Dr. S. Weir Mitchell (Chapter 2), no drug can reach the cause back of each disease. There is one other reason God ideally wants us to trust Him alone. He tells us in Isaiah 42:8: "I am the Lord: that is my name; and my glory will I not give to another...." Thus, when we use the Lord *plus* other things, His glory *can* be diminished.

Death, the "Terminal Illness"

There is another objection to healing. Occasionally someone says, "Everyone since Adam's fall has to die, so we cannot prevent the terminal illness." We have had people ask the question, "Do you believe that someone can live forever?" These are two ways of expressing the same concern. This is a very important question and one that must be answered. There have been several attempts to answer it.

Some people say that, since we all have to die, we cannot necessarily be healed at any particular time. This answer actually prevents the investigation into divine healing. We need to see how to determine if an illness is, indeed, the terminal one for an individual. The Bible does teach that sin came into the world by Adam's sin (Romans 5:12) and that death came by sin. There are many factors to consider, however.

Enoch (Genesis 5:22) and Elijah (2 Kings 2:11) went to be with the Lord without passing through the normal processes of disease and dying. We should note parenthetically that the author of Hebrews states that Enoch was translated by faith (11:5) and implies that his faith pleased God. Very few of us reach the heights of faith that Enoch reached. So we see that some people have died or have gone to be with the Lord without going through a disease or death process. Some people have reported very old believers announcing that "it is time for me to go home," and then just peacefully dying. Some people believe that we do not ever have to die from disease, that we can just get old and quit breathing (*e.g.*, Kenneth Hagin teaches this).[1] I feel that this is an oversimplification.

It is true that the Bible never says that death has to come by disease. To say that we do not have to die from illness really begs the question, however. Since illness and its end product, death, came into the world by Adam's sin, death due to illness and death due to the body's getting old and tired and ceasing to function are very akin to each other. Both are results of the fall, and Satan works in both. (He comes *only* to steal, kill, and destroy.)

What is really at stake in healing is whether we allow Satan to kill a person before the time allotted for his life. Job indicates that God intends us to die only when we are "ripe" like a shock of grain (Job 5:26)—*i.e.*, when we have lived long enough to complete what God put us on earth to do.

A general rule, unless God specifically reveals to us that we have fewer or more years, is that He, during this period of time, has given us seventy years—eighty in cases of special strength (Psalm 90:10). A life span shorter than that *may* be shorter than the amount allotted. Watchman Nee suggests that for a person under seventy years of age we wage spiritual battle in prayer for that person's life: "Now we are not suggesting that everybody must live to be at least seventy, for we cannot encroach on God's sovereignty like that; but in case we receive no registration of a shorter period, **let us accept this number as standard and repulse any earlier departure. By standing on the Word of God we will see victory** [my emphasis]." [2]

Moses died when he was 120 years old, but he had the strength, eyesight, and vigor of a man much younger (Deuteronomy 34:5-7). Moses died, not because he was ill, but because of his disobedience to God (citation). Moses' lifespan, therefore, was shorter than God's will for him.

Thus, we would encourage every believer to pray for healing, and we would encourage believers to agree in prayer regarding the healing of another believer. Those prayers should be continued unless God indicates that He has determined to take that person "home." A few times, when praying for a believer's healing, we have experienced God's letting us know that the person's time to depart has come. We also know of several people who have realized that their lifespan was complete. In these cases in which God has revealed that He will not be healing an individual, He is actually giving a *rhema* concerning that person.

To summarize, we believe that for a person, especially a person under 70 or 80 years of age, we should battle in prayer for that person's healing. When we do that, we find that God is gracious to let us know if He is not going to heal that person. At that point we can cease praying for healing. We can also pray for healing for an older person, but we need to keep in mind that that person may well have completed the work that God has for him to do.

Lack of Universal Healing

We need to address one other aspect in thinking about some people's resistance to healing. Occasionally, someone says, "Not everyone gets healed, so it must not be something upon which we can count." The response for this statement is to say, "God provided salvation for everyone, but not all believe and are saved. Similarly, He provided healing for each believer, but not all believers avail themselves of this benefit."

Connected with this is a very unfortunate fact. Sometimes people are jealous of someone's healing if they or a close friend or relative did not receive healing. In Chapter 6 we told Susan's story of healing. Her Bible teacher told her, "My mother was not healed; she was a good Christian; you must not have been healed by God." Some people told her that she must have gone into Christian Science doctrine. It is a sad commentary on the Christian fellowship that not all rejoice when God heals another brother or sister.

We have answered the most commonly used objections to accepting that God has provided healing for all believers. We have seen that it is God's will for His children to walk in health and victory. We must not let Satan rob us of the benefits that Jesus has won for us.

[1] Kenneth Hagin, *Seven Things You Should Know About Divine Healing* (Tulsa: Faith Library Publications, 1995), pp. 21-24.

[2] Watchman Nee, *The Spiritual Man*, Vol. III (New York: Christian Fellowship Publishers, Inc., 1968), p. 219.

9
When God Does Not Heal

There are several reasons in individual circumstances why God does not heal. Some are easy to understand; others are much more difficult. We will begin with the easier ones.

Sin

The simplest (and, I suspect, the most frequent) reason why God does not heal is due to sin. There is a direct relationship between sin and death or disease, as we mentioned in Chapter 8.

In Old Testament times God disciplined the Israelites with disease and/or death for their sins. Thus, a fire from the Lord devoured Nadab and Abihu, two of the sons of Aaron, when they offered strange fire before the Lord (Leviticus 10:1-2). The earth opened up and swallowed Korah and his comrades alive who had rebelled against Moses and Aaron, and fire from the Lord consumed the 250 men who offered incense (Numbers 16:1-35). God indicated that some sickness would follow anti-Semitism: "…[the Lord] will lay them [all sickness] upon all those who hate thee" (Deuteronomy 7:15). In Deuteronomy 28:60 sickness is coupled with sin, and David indicates in Psalm 51 that his terrible illnesses and bodily complaints are due directly to his sin.

In the church age God also disciplines us with disease—and occasionally death. Paul writes that many in the Corinthian church were sick and had died (are sleeping) because of unconfessed sin at the communion table (1 Corinthians 11:30). When a believer in the church in Corinth persisted in the sin of incest (1 Corinthians 5:1-5), Paul commanded his body to be turned over to Satan that his soul might be saved. Thus, he was turned over for death because of his sin (see further discussion below). In 2 Corinthians 2:4-11, we see that this sentence of death was commuted because he repented. In fact, Paul had to chide the Corinthians because they were so self-righteous that they refused to take him back into fellowship!

When a believer dies because of sin, we say that he has committed the "sin unto death." This terminology comes from 1 John 5:16-17: "If any man see his brother sin a sin which is not unto death, he shall ask, and he shall give him life for them that sin not unto death. There is a sin unto death; I do not say that he shall pray for it. All unrighteousness is sin, and there is a sin not unto death." John indicates that some sins in our lives are such that God decrees our death as a result. He is very clear, however, that not all sin has this sentence of death. John indicates that we can pray for a person who does not commit the sin unto death, and life (opposite of death and its companion, illness) will result. This shows that sin is linked with illness and death. We noted in the last chapter that Moses' death was due to sin.

Sin, of course, can be mental attitude sins, sins of the tongue, or overt action sins. Because we do not know the heart of a person, we cannot judge whether a person is ill or dies because of sin, apart from revelation from God. God's judgment on sin is almost always different from ours. Isaiah tells us that God's thoughts are higher than ours and that His ways are higher than ours, even to the degree that heaven is higher than the earth (Isaiah 55:9). A list of the seven sins God hates most is in Proverbs 6:16-19. Three are mental attitude; three are sins of the tongue; only murder is an overt action. (See fuller discussion in Chapter 10)

On some occasions repentance causes God to annul the death sentence. Two examples of this are King David and the believer in the church at Corinth. Appendix B gives some examples in the Bible of persons who commit the sin unto death and the results of that sin.

James addresses the "sin unto death," saying that the "prayer of faith shall save the sick, and the Lord shall raise him up; and if he have committed sins, they shall be forgiven him. Confess your faults one to another, and pray one for another, that ye may be healed" (James 5:15-16a). Thus, he implies that if one has not committed sin unto death, confession of sin and prayer will result in healing. We see clearly, therefore, that lack of healing *may* be a result of sin. In its most severe form it is the sin unto death.

Paul makes it clear that this is *not* the unpardonable sin when he deals with the believer in the Corinthian church. We can think of the description that Paul gives in 1 Corinthians 5:5 almost as a graph, or picture. He says that the church is to deliver the believer to Satan for the destruction of the flesh (or body) that his spirit may have eternal salvation. The picture is that of a believer falling down, down, down. It is as though, *if he were left alone*, he could slip out of his saved position because of his continued sin. God, however, commands him to be turned over to Satan to destroy his body (that is, to kill him), thus stopping him short of that line and saving his spirit for the day of the Lord. This does not argue for a believer losing his salvation because God, in fact, would have stopped the process of sin in this case by having Satan destroy his body. (This actually did not have to go to this point, because the believer did repent; but the point is that God was intervening in the believer's life to see that he did not fall away from salvation.)

In Chapter 10 we will see that one should confess every known sin, and thus be cleansed from all unrighteousness, before seeking healing.

Unbelief

Closely related to sin's being a reason that God sometimes does not heal is unbelief.

We see this in the case of Moses. When the Israelites complained and murmured because of lack of water at Kadesh, Moses sinned and disobeyed God by smiting the rock twice when God told him only to speak to it. Yet God tells Moses, **"Because ye believed me not**, to sanctify me in the eyes of the children of Israel..."** (our emphasis). Thus, in this case, disobedience is linked to disbelief. This, in turn, was the direct cause of Moses' death before he could enter the Promised Land.

A more frequent type of unbelief is that of the modern-day church. Most of the people in the church today do not believe that God will heal them; thus, they never get healed. Some have never been told what the Bible teaches about healing; worse, some have been taught that the Bible teaches that healing is *not* for the church today. In the forty years I had been in evangelical, Bible-believing, Bible teaching churches and the twenty-five years Bruce had been in them, *neither of us had ever once heard a sermon or teaching on healing that indicated that healing is available for all believers.* Jesus Himself was limited in performing miracles in Nazareth because of unbelief (see Matthew 13:58 and Mark 6:5-6), although He did perform a few "private healings."

Since the church has not taught healing as a rule, many Christians are very confused. Even when a Christian learns that God does heal, frequently there is a lot of unbelief mixed with the faith. There is one person with whom we talked over a period of a couple of years. Martin had struggled with depression for years. Although the onset of his depression probably had a clinical reason, he began to see that God could heal him from the grip of the depression. When he was depressed, his family life was impacted to a great degree. He received a personal *rhema*, showing him how God wanted him to break out of the depression cycle. God also began to open Scripture after Scripture showing him that He wanted to heal him. Almost immediately after receiving his *rhema*, doubt crept in, and he began to rationalize all that the Lord had shown him. He went from counselor to counselor, trying to find someone who could help him resolve his problems. He began asking, "Don't you think God can use medicine to heal me?" Of course, God can use anything, but God does not need medicine to heal. As we discussed in Chapter 8, God refuses to share his glory with another (Isaiah 42:8; 48:1). As Martin dwelled more and more on what God could not do (heal without medicine), his unbelief eventually led him to fail to receive healing. As a result, he is on multiple medications, some with side effects, and all probably for life. Unbelief can keep a person bound in illness.

Wrong Geographical Location

Sometimes God does not heal if a person is in the wrong place geographically. This is closely related to the section on unbelief above. This factor limited Jesus' ministry. Matthew 13:58 and Mark 6:5-6, cited above, indicate that Jesus could do no "mighty" work in Nazareth, His hometown because of its unbelief. He did, however, perform a few healing miracles, apparently in a very low-key fashion.

Jesus' healing of the blind man from Bethsaida is even more revealing. Bethsaida was a city which Jesus had condemned for its unbelief: "Then began he to upbraid the cities wherein most of his mighty works were done, because they repented not: Woe unto thee, Chorazin! woe unto thee, Bethsaida! for if the mighty works, which were done in you, had been done in Tyre and Sidon, they would have repented long ago in sackcloth and ashes. But I say unto you, It shall be more tolerable for Tyre and Sidon at the day of judgment, than for you" (Matthew 11:20-22—see also Luke 10:13). When some people brought the blind man from Bethsaida to Jesus, Jesus took him by the hand and led him out of the town, where He healed him. Then he told him not to go back into the town and not to tell anyone in the town (Mark 8:22-26). Thus, that particular healing apparently could not be done in the town that did not believe.

How can one know if this problem is keeping him from being healed? We would suggest that, if one has sought the Lord for healing and has received no other answer, he should consider it. One should ask some questions:

1. Does the Holy Spirit seem stifled in this area?
2. Is there an air of oppression about the area?
3. Do the churches in the area see healings?
4. Do the churches in the area encourage members to call for the elders for anointing with oil and prayer for healing?

These kinds of questions can reveal a problem in the area. We have lived in at least two areas with such problems. When Bruce was moving to one of these, severe attacks in the spirit realm hit him when he turned off the main road to another road leading to this town. We later learned that one of the leading evangelists of the twentieth century had long ago seen this place as very dead spiritually and even antithetic to the Gospel.

In the other area, there was an obvious oppression in the area. We once had a visitor who remarked that there seemed to be oppression when he drove into the town. An unbeliever in the town remarked to us that the town seemed "depressed." We learned later that a major spiritualist group was headquartered there.

It may not be practical for one to move, but he may have to seek help outside the area. He certainly would have to have support as he stands in his healing from outside. When it is practical, the person might be helped by moving to an area where there is more faith operating.

Satanic or Demonic Bondage

There is a type of illness and/or infirmity that has a Satanic or demonic cause. Sometimes a person can receive healing from this type of illness in the normal ways—*i.e.*, laying on of hands, prayer of faith, or miracle. At other times, however, the root problem must be addressed. Thus, one must discover the "door" through which the Satanic or demonic entered, renounce it, confess any sin associated with it, and close the door of access. Only then can healing come.

Although it is beyond the scope of this book to do an exhaustive study on the demonic, there are many good books available. One of the best is Derek Prince's *They Shall Expel Demons*, coupled with his *Blessing or Curse: You Can Choose*.

Many of the illnesses that Jesus healed were of this sort. Jesus saw a woman who was "bowed together, and could in no wise lift herself up" (Luke 13:11). Today we would probably recognize such a woman as having rheumatoid arthritis. Jesus, however, had to recognize that it was Satan who had bound her and had to rebuke the spirit of infirmity in order to heal her. He "said unto her, Woman, thou art loosed from thine infirmity. And he laid his hands on her; and immediately she was made straight, and glorified God" (vs. 12b-13). When the ruler of the synagogue protested this healing on the Sabbath day, Jesus said, "...ought not this woman...whom Satan hath bound, lo, these eighteen years, be loosed from this bond on the sabbath day?" (v. 16). Thus the Lord refers to this healing, not as a healing as such, but as a loosing from the bond that Satan had tied.

I experienced an infirmity of this sort. We had a special worship service at the church we were attending. At one point the pastor asked for people to come to the front, kneel, and pray for revival. I felt that I should participate. My left knee was almost fully recovered from pains from a knee injury I had suffered the previous year; but I leaned more on the right knee since the left was newly recovered from the injury Late in the proceedings the pastor asked people to lay hands on those nearby them and to pray for them. Later that evening and the next day my right knee was painful. I attributed that to being in an awkward position in the kneeling, but I thought that God would not let the kneeling hurt me, since I was worshipping Him.

As time progressed, the knee got worse. It became very painful. We just did not understand why God was not healing the knee. I had confessed every known sin in my life; I believed that God had healed me by Christ's atonement; I prayed to receive the healing, thanked God, and tried to walk in that healing. But there was no real improvement.

Finally, after about two months Bruce felt that we had to pray through to victory on the knee. Many times, as we prayed, Bruce got an image of something's being wrong with my going down to the front of the church that night. I examined my heart for motives; I asked God to reveal the thoughts and intents of my heart; but I could find nothing amiss. Bruce kept telling me that he thought I needed to repent; I told him that I would if I were convicted of something, but I had not been. We did not doubt that Bruce was being given a correct revelation, but we could not see how it all fit together. I was convinced that there was nothing wrong *per se* in my going down.

Finally, one night while we were praying, as the picture of something being wrong with that night kept coming back to Bruce, he asked me if anyone laid hands on me, and I said that two people had. Suddenly, like a flash, I knew that that was what was wrong. I had read a passage in Derek Prince's book *They Shall Expel Demons*, relating an experience that his wife Ruth had when she was a new believer in which there was a service with casual laying on of hands and in which she was given a spirit of arthritis.

I repented of the casual laying on of hands and asked God to close any door to Satan that I might have opened. Immediately, the knee was 90% better. We praised God for the breakthrough. I resolved to walk in that victory. We saw a steady improvement in the pain and malfunction of that knee. As we prayed following that night, Bruce did not see the picture of that service anymore. Thus, we feel that the legal opening for Satan was closed, and that God healed me. I stood in that healing and gradually saw the symptoms line up with the healing.

The excerpt from Derek Prince's book *They Shall Expel Demons* stresses the importance of taking care in the laying on of hands:

> Laying hands on a person in prayer is not just a picturesque religious ritual. It can be a powerful spiritual experience, a temporary interaction between two spirits through which supernatural power is released. Normally the power flows from the one laying on hands to the one on whom hands are laid, but at times it can flow the other way.
> The power may do either good or evil. It may emanate from the Holy Spirit or from a demon, depending on the one from whom it flows. For this reason Paul established certain safeguards. "Do not lay hands on

anyone hastily," he wrote, "nor share in other people's sins; keep yourself pure" (1 Timothy 5:22). In other words, be careful with whom you allow your spirit to interact!

The laying on of hands should be done reverently and prayerfully. Any person participating should make sure he or she is not thereby, in Paul's words, sharing in another person's sins.

It is a mistake to turn a group of people loose and encourage them to lay hands indiscriminately on one another. The following brief testimony from Ruth illustrates the danger:

> In 1971 I was attending a charismatic meeting, and the speaker asked people to stand if they wanted prayer for healing, I had a bad cold, so I stood. He then instructed people seated nearby to lay their hands on us and pray for our healing. Four or five prayed for me.
>
> When I awoke the next morning, my cold was better—but my fingers were all curled up and stiff and hurting. Immediately I thought, *Someone with arthritis laid hands on me lost night!* I renounced the spirit of arthritis, and within five minutes all the symptoms were gone.
>
> I was a very young believer, less than one year old, and I have been so grateful to God for teaching me then to be careful who lays hands on me.[1]

We have attended far too many services in which a minister asks people to lay hands on an individual without knowing the state of the people who are laying their hands on the person. Thus, when God does not appear to heal, one should examine himself to see if there is a possibility of a demonic cause. As mentioned earlier, I am not dealing with this area in this book. There are several good books on the subject.

Refusal of Healing

One of the seemingly strangest reasons for a person not to receive healing is for that person to refuse it. We might be tempted to say, "No one would turn down healing," but sadly this is not the case. We have had experience with several people who, for various reasons, refused healing.

We have shown throughout our discussion of healing that there are many parallels between the healing and the salvation processes. In Chapter 3, when we discussed the faith principle, we learned that, since faith is the "currency of the kingdom," some of the same principles work in any area in which faith is needed. We all probably know personally or have heard accounts of people who have refused salvation.

For example, in Bruce's family, after Bruce's father became a believer, he tried to evangelize all his family and friends. When he was talking to an elderly relative, the relative turned down salvation, saying, "My [deceased] wife and I had an agreement that we would go to the same place, so I cannot break that agreement."

We have heard Ben Haden, former pastor of First Presbyterian Church in Chattanooga and founder of *Changed Lives*, tell of visiting a man who had only an hour to live. Rev. Haden asked him if he knew if he had only one hour to live. The man replied in the affirmative. Rev. Haden then explained salvation and asked him to accept God's free gift. The man said that he could not because he would have to admit that he had been wrong all his life.

Since we know of cases in which people have turned down God's free gift of salvation, apparently knowing what they are doing, it should not surprise us that some people will turn down healing. There are many reasons for this. Some people have become comfortable in their surroundings with their illness. They might like the attention, the fact that they are not expected to work, or a number of other factors. Sometimes they know the spiritual battle that they will have to wage if they pray for healing. They are tired and do not wish to battle any longer. In a related way some people think that they can receive a "miracle" healing; when they learn that they must battle, sometimes for years, to get and to keep their healing, they lose heart and choose not to receive the healing. At any rate, this is one of the saddest reasons people do not receive healing.

We counseled a young man, David, for many months on a weekly basis. He was referred to us by a friend who sensed that God was working with him and letting him know that He wanted to heal him. David had multiple medical problems, some of which had no cure. His condition was not fatal, but it caused him severe infirmity. He was able to do very little work. Prior to our introduction David had been led to Isaiah 53 and to the reference to it in 1 Peter 2:24: "Who his own self bare our sins in his own body on the tree, that we, being dead to sins, should live unto righteousness: by whose stripes ye were healed." This friend correctly perceived that God had been working with him and that he was ready for healing. We spent several weeks getting acquainted and hearing all the details of his 20-year medical history. We began showing him more Scriptures to reinforce what God had been teaching him. Eventually, he began to realize that, if he were healed, he would probably be expected to work more, perhaps even full time. He also began to realize that the dynamics of his relationship with his extended family would change. He had become comfortable in the particular relationships in his family.

At that point he rejected the healing, not wanting to disturb the pattern of his life. He is now facing more surgery and probable increased infirmity.

We related in Chapter 6 how our friend Sally was healed. She also fell into this trap. At the time of her healing there were a couple of life-style changes that she knew God wanted her to make. These would have involved intense spiritual struggle. She was very fatigued—both from her illness and from the spiritual battle to that point. She decided not to "keep" her healing; the battle was not worth it to her. She told me, "There are worse things than dying. I'll be waiting for you up there." Interestingly enough, about the time of the onset of her illness, God gave her a dream that told her how she could overcome the disease. She dreamed that Satan was chasing her and that she was running hard. Satan was gaining on her, and she did not know what to do. She suddenly realized the solution. She stopped and shouted to him, "Be gone, in the name of the Lord Jesus Christ." And Satan left her alone. She and we believed that the Lord was letting her know ahead of time that the Lord Jesus could defeat this illness that Satan was placing on her.

God does not normally override our free will, either for salvation or for healing. Thus, if a person decides not to be healed, usually he is not healed.

Unknown Causes

There are some cases in which the person apparently has faith for healing. Prayer has gone up, and there is no healing. There is apparently no unconfessed sin, nor has the person apparently committed the sin unto death. There appears to be no possibility of a demonic cause for the illness, nor does there appear to be a geographic problem.

In these cases we have to say we just do not know what God is doing. God is God, after all, and His ways are above our ways, and His thoughts are above our thoughts. Deuteronomy 29:29 is *apropos* in this situation: "The secret *things belong* unto the LORD our God: but those *things which are* revealed *belong* unto us and to our children for ever, that *we* may do all the words of this law" (Deuteronomy 29:29).

Jeremiah asks how the clay can object to the potter's work: "The word which came to Jeremiah from the LORD, saying, Arise, and go down to the potter's house, and there I will cause thee to hear my words. Then I went down to the potter's house, and, behold, he wrought a work on the wheels. And the vessel that he made of clay was marred in the hand of the potter: so he made it again another vessel, as seemed good to the potter to make *it*. Then the word of the LORD came to me, saying, O house of Israel, cannot I do with you as this potter? saith the LORD. Behold, as the clay *is* in the potter's hand, so *are* ye in mine hand, O house of Israel" (Jeremiah 18:1-6).

Paul echoes this thought: "Nay but, O man, who art thou that repliest against God? Shall the thing formed say to him that formed *it*, Why hast thou made me thus? Hath not the potter power over the clay, of the same lump to make one vessel unto honour, and another unto dishonour" (Romans 9:20-21).

I personally feel that we can never reach a state of having all illness gone. When we are saved from our sin, we still have trouble with sins as long as we are in our sinful bodies. John tells us in his first epistle that we lie if we say we have no sin (1 John 1:8). In a similar way we will always have trouble with illness, one of the products of sin. We can appropriate God's healing much more than we do at the present time, but there will always be times when our sinful bodies just cannot seem to win the victory. Nevertheless, we should press in and try for the ideal.

We would give one caution at this point. **It is important not to judge a person who has not received his healing.** We do not know what is going on inside that person or what the Lord is doing with him. Unless God gives us a *rhema* for that person, we cannot presume to judge.

God refuses to let us put Him in a box. We should never think that we have the workings of God figured out like some mathematics formula. When we do not understand what God is doing, we simply bow our heads, thank God for being God, and humbly submit ourselves to His workings.

[1]Derek Prince, *They Shall Expel Demons*, (Grand Rapids: Chosen Books, 1998), pp. 109-110.

10
Steps to Take for Personal Healing

We have established that part of the character of God is His unchanging nature as the Eternal Healer. We have seen that the Bible teaches that complete healing was provided for the believer in the atonement of our Lord. We have developed the "faith principle" and have seen how to take the doctrine of healing and apply it to a particular individual. We have looked at various methods God uses to heal, at the spiritual gift of healing, at some objections to healing, and at reasons God sometimes does not heal.

Now we need to look at some practical advice for obtaining healing based on the material in the previous chapters. When a person becomes ill—whether it be a seemingly small cold or a major, life-threatening disease—the steps to take for healing are very straightforward.

Call for the Elders of the Church

As we have noted, James (5:14-15) gives us a command: we are to call for the elders of the church to anoint the individual and pray for healing. One might feel self-conscious about doing this for a "simple cold," but many churches have healing services during the week when one can approach the leadership of the church for this ministry. As we have noted, the language in the original does not allow for options. The original language makes it clear that it is a command for a one-time action for healing for a particular disease. Thus, the believer needs to have the elders pray and anoint him one time; then, he is to praise the Lord and rejoice in his healing.

Confess All Known Sin

Confess all known sin. The importance of this cannot be overstressed. There is more to this step than meets the eye. We are told very clearly, "If I regard iniquity in my heart, the Lord will not hear me" (Psalm 66:18). We should note that this Scripture tells us to examine our hearts for iniquity; this is quite different from just knowing in our minds that there is a problem. Solomon tells us, "The sacrifice of the wicked is an abomination to the Lord, but the prayer of the upright is his delight" (Proverbs 15:8), and Isaiah says to the inhabitants of Judah who were far from the Lord, "...when ye make many prayers, I will not hear. Your hands are full of blood" (Isaiah 1:15).

Thus, before we pray any prayer for healing, we must approach God upright and without iniquity. How can we do this? Certainly, we never reach sinless perfection in this life. John tells us, "If we say that we have no sin, we deceive ourselves, and the truth is not in us....If we say that we have not sinned, we make him a liar, and his word is not in us" (1 John 1:8,10). John, however, gives us the solution: "If we confess our sins, he is faithful and just to forgive us our sins, and to cleanse us from all unrighteousness" (1 John 1:9). Thus, if we confess the sins of which we are aware, God forgives us from them and also cleanses us from all the sins, or unrighteousness, about which we are not aware.

This is extremely important. This does not involve just a quick, "Lord, forgive me." It involves intense soul searching. Jeremiah tells us that "[t]he heart is deceitful above all things, and desperately wicked; who can know it?" (Jeremiah 17:9). We cannot, therefore, even know sometimes what wickedness is in our hearts. How then are we to discover this and confess it? Jeremiah answers that question, "I, the Lord, search the heart, I test the conscience, even to give every man according to his ways, and according to the fruit of his doings" (Jeremiah 17:10). David indicates much the same principle: "Search me, O God, and know my heart; try me, and know my thoughts; And see if there be any wicked way in me, and lead me in the way everlasting" (Psalm 139:23-24).

We must learn in our spirits how to apply Hebrews 4:12: "For the word of God *is* quick, and powerful, and sharper than any twoedged sword, piercing even to the dividing asunder of soul and spirit, and of the joints and marrow, and *is* a discerner of the thoughts and intents of the heart." Only the Word of God applied can perform this kind of "surgery."

We see, then, that we need God's great "searchlight" to look into the depths of our hearts and reveal to us the wickedness there. Then, we can make the proper confession. The word translated *confess* from 1 John 1:9 (quoted above) simply means "agree with." We are being asked to agree with God that the sin He shows us is indeed sin.

Another factor to consider is that God's list of most hated sins rarely matches ours. Again, as Isaiah tells us, "For my thoughts *are* not your thoughts, neither *are* your ways my ways, saith the LORD. For *as* the heavens are higher than the earth, so are my ways higher than your ways, and my thoughts than your thoughts" (Isaiah 55:8-9). We cannot even begin to think as God thinks.

I enjoy a little exercise when I am teaching. I like to distribute pens and paper and ask people to list what they think are the worst sins. Many tend to be listed every time—murder, adultery, violence. Occasionally someone names pride. God tells us the seven he hates the most in Proverbs 6:16-19: "These six *things* doth the LORD hate: yea, seven *are* an abomination unto him: A proud look, a lying tongue, and hands that shed innocent blood, An heart that deviseth wicked imaginations, feet that be swift in running to mischief, A false witness *that* speaketh lies, and he that soweth discord among brethren." Only one sin is an overt sin: murder. Three are sins of the tongue, and three are mental attitude sins.

In addition, we have to understand how the Hebrew language indicates the superlative degree of a word, indicating the most extreme of that word. (For example, if we want to say that someone is pretty, we say *pretty*; but if we want to indicate that a person has that trait more than anyone else in a certain group, we use the superlative. We would say, "She is the prettiest girl in the school.") In English most words form the superlative by adding *est* to the word or using the word *most* with the word (*i.e.*, most beautiful). One of the ways of showing this in Hebrew is to say "the [word] of the [word]." *King of Kings*, therefore, means the "most kingly" king in the world.

Another way of showing the superlative in Hebrew is used in these verses in Proverbs. The formula "[a certain number], yea, [that number plus one]" indicates that the last named is the one with the most of that characteristic. Therefore, when Solomon said, "These six things doth the Lord hate: yea seven are an abomination unto him," he was indicating that the seventh is the one that God hates most. How many of us would put sowing discord among brethren as the worst sin? It is true that God's thoughts are so far above our thoughts we can scarcely understand them. That is why God Himself must search our hearts, deep in our spirits, to reveal to us the sins that are present. Once these are brought to our attention, we can confess them and receive cleansing and prepare ourselves further for our healing. It is very helpful to pray the prayer from Psalm 139 quoted above.

Forgive All Trespasses

Related to the confessing of known sin in our lives is the fact that we must forgive anyone who has ever wronged us. Many people in deliverance ministries have stated that lack of forgiving those who have wronged them keeps more people from victory than any other one factor. Derek Prince, for example, affirms this in *They Shall Expel Demons.*

Jesus told us that if we do not forgive others' trespasses against us, the Father will not forgive us, "For if ye forgive men their trespasses, your heavenly Father will also forgive you: But if ye forgive not men their trespasses, neither will your Father forgive your trespasses" (Matthew 6: 14-15). We tend not to take this admonition seriously, but there is no rationale to disregard these words of the Lord; we cannot choose to believe some of His words and ignore others.

Jesus indicates that we cannot even worship God if we have unresolved problems with a brother: "Therefore if thou bring thy gift to the altar, and there rememberest that thy brother hath ought against thee; Leave there thy gift before the altar, and go thy way; first be reconciled to thy brother, and then come and offer thy gift" (Matthew 5:23-24).

Holding grudges and lack of forgiveness are big obstacles for healing or for any other kind of progress in our Christian lives.

Pray the Prayer of Faith Using a *Rhema*

Once we have confessed all known sin, including the sin of lack of forgiveness, we are ready to pray the prayer of faith.

We can simply pray this prayer ourselves, using Scriptures that God has impressed upon us, and ask our Father for healing as we discussed in Chapter 3. This is the point at which one must have a *rhema* from God. Faith cannot be "whipped up" out of nothing. If we do not have a *rhema* at this point, we must go into prayer and Bible meditation and not stop until we have a *rhema* from God. It is helpful to meditate on Scriptures that deal with healing.

This point cannot be overstressed. **To proceed confidently in faith, one must have a *rhema*.** In trying to help various people, we have seen a problem in this area. Some people have learned that they must have this *rhema*. They will search the Scriptures and find a verse that speaks about healing. They will take this verse and say, "This is my *rhema*." That is not what constitutes a *rhema*. That is an example of hope; they are hoping that this verse will "work." This is very close to the groups who encourage one to "name it and claim it." A person names it (designates his own *rhema*) and then claims it (states that this means God will heal him). A person should remember that *rhema* means "utterance" or "word," as in a word from God. One must be very sure that the particular Scripture was given to him by God. We have discussed the ways in which this word can come—by the still, small voice, usually when meditating on the Scripture; when a Scripture just "jumps out," showing that God is calling one's attention to that word; with an "inner knowing," again often when meditating on the Scripture; and by God's speaking directly to the individual, sometimes in an audible voice. (Great care must be made to make sure that the *rhema* comes from God; Satan loves to give us false hope and thus circumvent God's working.) When a person gets the *rhema* showing that God wants to heal him at this point, he can take that word, stand on it strongly, and persist in battle until the healing comes. He has a word with which he can stare down all the foes of Satan—in the power of God.

Occasionally, a *rhema* can come from a source outside the individual. In those cases, however, the person usually has to believe the word and then exercise faith. An example is that of Naaman, the captain of the army of the king of Syria. He sought healing from his leprosy from God through the prophet Elisha (2 Kings 5:1-27). Elisha told him to wash in the Jordan River seven times, and his leprosy would be healed (that was his *rhema*). He protested at first and then decided to follow the instructions, and then he was healed. This example also shows another principle. Naaman was told to wash in the river; this could be likened to someone's being told to use some medicine or to have some surgery. The important thing is to hear from God and to follow His instructions completely—whether to stand in faith for healing, whether to take medicine, or whether to have a procedure like surgery or chemotherapy.

Get the Agreement of Other Believers

The prayer of faith may be prayed by the ill individual alone, or other believers may agree in prayer with the person, as we also discussed in Chapter 6. Even if the ill individual initially prays the prayer of faith by himself, it greatly helps in the battle that that person will almost certainly have to fight with Satan to have other believers agreeing in prayer about the healing. The power of the prayer when there is more than one person involved is not counted arithmetically, but it increases geometrically. Leviticus 26:8 tells us: "And five of you shall chase an hundred, and an hundred of you shall put ten thousand to flight...." It is very helpful to have this added power in the struggle.

Admit No Doubt within the Circle of Prayer

One cautionary note needs to be made at this point. It is extremely important that the "inner circle" that is praying for the healing include **no one** who is doubting or wavering. James cautioned us against having this spirit present in any prayer of faith: "But let him ask in faith, nothing wavering. For he that wavereth is like a wave of the sea driven with the wind and tossed. For let not that man think that he shall receive any thing of the Lord. A double minded man *is* unstable in all his ways" (James 1:6-8). Faith is the "currency of the kingdom" (see Hebrews 11: 6), and there can be no compromise in this area.

God may not answer a prayer for healing because he cannot answer the prayer of a prayer partner who is wavering. It may seem hard to exclude a family member or close friend, but it could literally be a matter of life and death. One should choose his prayer partners carefully. We personally know of situations in which the person did not receive healing because a prayer "partner" was either praying against the person or praying in unbelief.

Confess the Healing and Maintain This Confession

As we discussed earlier, we must confess our healing and maintain this confession. We have heard of people who received God's healing and who had to maintain the confession in the face of *seemingly* no results. There are people who have had to do this for as long as a year, seeing no healing in the natural. But, when they "saw" with their spiritual eyes and maintained their confession, eventually the symptoms lined up with their confession. Paul tells us that we have a God "who giveth life to the dead, and calleth those things which are not, as though they were" (Romans 4:17b). We must agree (confess) with God in calling our healing accomplished before we see the symptoms line up with the confession.

This step is one in which the importance of the *rhema* is clear. When Satan tries to attack, when the symptoms are contrary to the healing, or when there is no visible progress, one can remain absolutely firm in "calling those things which are not as though they were" if he has a *rhema*. One can stand on God's promises in the face of *any* attack or adverse circumstance. The importance of having a *rhema* cannot be overemphasized.

Praise the Lord

Possibly the most important part of our healing is to praise (and worship) the Lord. We should begin to praise the Lord with our prayer of faith and never cease to give Him praise. He alone is worthy of all praise, honor, and glory. He has told us, "I am the Lord: that is my name; and my glory will I not give to another, neither my praise to graven images" (Isaiah 42:8). Thus, He and He alone is to get the glory for our healing. Admonitions to praise the Lord abound in the Scriptures.

The writer of Hebrews exhorts us: "…let us offer the sacrifice of praise to God continually, that is, the fruit of our lips giving thanks to his name" (Hebrews 13:15). The Old Testament uses the two primary words for praise nearly three hundred times.

Following are only a few of the passages:

Praise ye the Lord. Praise the Lord, O my soul. While I live will I praise the Lord. I will sing praises unto my God while I have any being.
                              Psalm 146:1-2

Bless the Lord, O my soul, and all that is within me, bless his holy name.
                              Psalm 103:1

Praise ye the LORD. Praise God in his sanctuary: praise him in the firmament of his power. Praise him for his mighty acts: praise him according to his excellent greatness. Praise him with the sound of the trumpet: praise him with the psaltery and harp. Praise him with the timbrel and dance: praise him with stringed instruments and organs. Praise him upon the loud cymbals: praise him upon the high sounding cymbals. Let every thing that hath breath praise the LORD. Praise ye the LORD.

Psalm 150

I will bless the Lord at all times; his praise shall continually be in my mouth.

Psalm 34:1

Give unto the Lord the glory due unto his name; worship the Lord in the beauty of holiness.

Psalm 29:2

I will praise thee, O Lord, with my whole heart; I will show forth all thy marvelous works. I will be glad and rejoice in thee; I will sing praise to thy name, O thou Most High.

Psalm 9:1

O Lord, thou art my God; I will exalt thee, I will praise thy name; for thou hast done wonderful things; thy counsels of old are faithfulness and truth.

Isaiah 25:1

The picture of Israel restored in the last days is one full of praise: "The voice of joy, and the voice of gladness; the voice of the bridegroom, and the voice of the bride; the voice of them who shall say, Praise the Lord of hosts; for the Lord is good; for his mercy endureth forever; and of those who shall bring the sacrifice of praise into the house of the Lord" (Jeremiah 33:11).

Finally, the picture we have of the throne room of God is that of creatures praising Jesus: "Thou art worthy, O Lord, to receive glory and honor and power; for thou hast created all things, and for thy pleasure they are and were created....And they sang a new song, saying, Thou art worthy to take the scroll, and to open its seals; for thou wast slain, and hast redeemed us to God by thy blood out of every kindred, and tongue, and people, and nation; And hast made us unto our God a kingdom of priests, and we shall reign on the earth" (Revelation 4:11; 5:9-10).

Many people have reported that praising the Lord seems to release something in the Heavenlies whereby the Lord begins to move on behalf of the sufferer. At a missions conference I was impressed by one of the missionaries who said, "We must teach God's people to praise Him." He added that we will have missions only during time; we will not have them in eternity. But praise will go on forever. When we praise God, we are "practicing" for eternity.

A Cautionary Note

Although we believe that God has provided for the healing of each believer, we cannot claim this provision in a flippant manner and proceed to live with disregard to the way God has made our bodies.

For example, overweight can cause added stress to our knees and other joints. We know the toll that tobacco or excessive alcohol intake causes to our bodies. Even extreme overwork can stress our bodies. Most of us have some area in which we have not taken care of our bodies perfectly. If there are problems in these areas, asking God to "heal" in an area we have abused may be rather like Satan's temptation of Christ, when he tempted Him to jump off the pinnacle of the temple and to ask God to save Him. Jesus answered that we should not tempt the Lord our God. Therefore, we should keep fit, get needed rest, and take care of the bodies the Lord has given us.

Paul's admonition to Timothy to "drink no longer water, but use a little wine for thy stomach's sake and thy frequent infirmities" (1Timothy 5:23) falls into this category. Water, in Paul's day, was frequently contaminated and could make someone ill. Thus, telling Timothy to guard against this assault on his body was simply a matter of treating his body with care.

In conclusion, we must in healing and in all other aspects of our lives submit ourselves "unto him that is able to do exceeding abundantly above all that we ask or think, according to the power that worketh in us, Unto him *be* glory in the church by Christ Jesus throughout all ages, world without end. Amen" (Ephesians 3:20-21).

Appendices

Appendix A

Individual Healed	Illness	Method	Scripture
Unnamed man	Leprosy	Touch of Jesus' hand	Matthew 8:1-4
Peter's mother-in-law	Fever	Jesus rebuked the fever, then took her by the hand, and lifted her up.	Matthew 8:14-15; Mark 1:29–31; Luke 4:38-39
2 unnamed men from Gadara	Demon possession	Spoken word	Matthew 8:28-34
2 unnamed men	Blindness	Jesus touched their eyes	Matthew 20:30-34
Unnamed man	Palsy (probably paralysis)	Sins forgiven, then word of healing spoken	Mark 2:1-12
Unnamed woman	Issue of blood	She touched Jesus' garment.	Mark 5:25–34
Daughter of Jairus	Death	Jesus took her by the hand and spoke the word.	Mark 5:21-24, 35–43
Many people in the land of Gennesaret	Various illnesses	Touching the border of Jesus' garments	Mark 6:53-56
Daughter of a Syrophenician woman	Unclean spirit	Spoken word—Jesus not present	Mark 7:24-30
Unnamed man	Blindness	Jesus spit on his eyes.	Mark 8:22-26
Many people in Galilee	Various illnesses	Jesus laid hands on them.	Luke 4:40-41

Individual healed	Illness	Method	Scripture
Centurion's servant	Ill on deathbed	Spoen word—Jesus not present	Luke 7:1-10
Widow's son	Death	Spoken word	Luke 7:11-15
Unnamed woman	Severe arthritis?	Spoken word	Luke 15:10-13
10 unnamed men	Leprosy	Jesus told them to go to the temple; they were healed as they went.	Luke 17:11-19
Servant of the high preist	Ear cut off	Jesus touch his ear.	Luke 22:50-51
Unnamed man	Impotent (could not walk)	Spoken word	John 5:2-9
Unnamed Man	Blind from birth	Jesus spat on the ground, made clay, put it on the eye of the man, and told him to wash in the pool of Siloam.	John 9:1-7
Lazarus	Death—more than four days	Spoken woord	John 11:1-44

Appendix B

Person(s)	Sin	Result	Scriptures
Nadab and Abihu	Offered strange fire	Death—fire from God	Leviticus 10:1-2
Israelites in wilderness	Unbelief	Death duing 40 years in desert before entering Promised Land	Numbers 14:26-34
Korah and others	Rebellion against God's authority	Death—swallowed alive by the earth and death by fire	Numbers 16:1-35
Moses and Aaron	Unbelief and disobedience to God's Word	Death before entering Promised Land	Numbers 20: 1-13; Deuteronomy 34:7
King Saul	Did not obey Word of God	Death and kingdom taken away from his family	1 Samuel 15:23; 28:18-19; 31:2-6
Uzzah	Touched Ark of the Covenant (disobeyed God)	Death	2 Samuel 6:6-7
King David	Adultery and murder	Death of son; David's death sentence commuted after repentance	2 Samuel 11; 12:5-14
Ananias and Sapphira	Testing (lying to the Holy Spirit)	Death	Acts 5:1-11
Believer in Corinthian church	Incest	Death sentence commuted after repentance	1 Corinthians 5:1-5; 2 Corinthians 2:4-11